Leadership Competencies for Clinical Managers

The Renaissance of Transformational Leadership

Anne M. Barker, EdD, RN
Associate Professor of Nursing
Sacred Heart University
Fairfield, Connecticut

Dori Taylor Sullivan, PhD, RN, CNA, CPHQ
Chair and Associate Professor of Nursing
Sacred Heart University
Fairfield, Connecticut

Michael J. Emery, PT, EdD
Chair and Associate Professor,
Department of Physical Therapy
and Human Movement Science
Sacred Heart University
Fairfield, Connecticut

JONES AND BARTLETT PUBLISHERS
Sudbury, Massachusetts
BOSTON   TORONTO   LONDON   SINGAPORE

World Headquarters
Jones and Bartlett Publishers
40 Tall Pine Drive
Sudbury, MA 01776
978-443-5000
info@jbpub.com
www.jbpub.com

Jones and Bartlett Publishers Canada
6339 Ormindale Way
Mississauga, Ontario L5V 1J2
Canada

Jones and Bartlett Publishers International
Barb House, Barb Mews
London W6 7PA
United Kingdom

Jones and Bartlett's books and products are available through most bookstores and online book-sellers. To contact Jones and Bartlett Publishers directly, call 800-832-0034, fax 978-443-8000, or visit our website, www.jbpub.com.

Substantial discounts on bulk quantities of Jones and Bartlett's publications are available to corporations, professional associations, and other qualified organizations. For details and specific discount information, contact the special sales department at Jones and Bartlett via the above contact information or send an email to specialsales@jbpub.com.

ISBN-13: 978-0-7637-4741-1
ISBN-10: 0-7637-4741-6

Production Credits

Acquisitions Editor: Kevin Sullivan
Associate Editor: Amy Sibley
Production Manager: Amy Rose
Production Editor: Susan Schultz
Marketing Manager: Emily Ekle
Manufacturing Buyer: Amy Bacus

Composition: GGS Book Services
Cover Design: Kristin E. Ohlin
Printing and Binding: Malloy, Inc.
Cover Image: © Photos.com
Cover Printing: Malloy, Inc.

Library of Congress Cataloging-in-Publication Data

Barker, Anne M.
 Leadership competencies for clinical managers : the renaissance of transformational leadership / Anne M. Barker, Dori Taylor Sullivan, Michael J. Emery.
 p. ; cm.
Includes bibliographical references and index.
 ISBN 0-7637-4741-6 (pbk.)
1. Health services administration. 2. Leadership. 3. Organizational change.
4. Organizational effectiveness.
 [DNLM: 1. Health Services Administration. 2. Personnel Management—methods.
3. Leadership. 4. Staff Development—methods. W 84.1 B255L 2006] I. Sullivan, Dori Taylor.
II. Emery, Michael J. III. Title.

 RA971.B272 2006
 362.1'068—dc22
 2005018120

6048

Printed in the United States of America
10 09 08 07 06   10 9 8 7 6 5 4 3 2

To Barbara, Neil, and Linda—
our partners in life and love

Table of Contents

Part One

**Chapter 3—Leadership IQ: An Evidence-Based
        Organizing Schema** **29**

Dori Taylor Sullivan and *Emmett C. Murphy*

**Chapter 4—Leadership Development Through Mentorship
        and Professional Development Planning** **45**

Anne M. Barker

Chapter 12—Human Resource Management Model **187**

Anne M. Barker

Chapter 13—Human Resource Management Strategies **213**

Anne M. Barker

Chapter 14—Marketing Initiatives **237**

Michael J. Emery

Part Three

Contributors

Emmett C. Murphy, PhD
Senior Fellow, LeadershipIQ.com
Former Chief and CEO
EC Murphy LLC/VHA

Linda Rusch, RN, MS, APN
Vice President Patient Care Services
Hunterdon Medical Center
Flemington, New Jersey

Colleen O. Smith, MSN, RN, CNAA
Vice President for Nursing
Middlesex Hospital
Middletown, Connecticut

Kathleen Stolzenberger, PhD, RN
Director of Research & Professional Development
Middlesex Hospital
Middletown, Connecticut

Foreword

Samuel B. Feitelberg

For anyone who aspires to assume and maintain a leadership role in the clinical disciplines there is nothing more essential than to understand and adopt leadership principles and practices in order to survive and prosper in today's chaotic health care environment. The emergence of a first-class work devoted to this essential subject is a welcome event.

For five decades texts, manuals, and workbooks devoted to the subject of leadership in single disciplines in a variety of health care settings have been crossing my desk. Now, it is refreshing to see a text that reaches out across the spectrum of clinical professions and presents content that draws them together through a compatible design.

It has required many years of practice for health care to move from single discipline teams working independently in the same environment to the arena of the multidisciplinary team working interdependently on behalf of the patient. As a result, the achievement of health care outcomes now relies on the insight, skill, and dedication of people working together. This builds a healthy and fruitful organizational climate and is the focus of the subject matter put forward in this excellent text.

The authors have ably assembled the theories, tools, and examples required for an effective education in leadership. Using transformational leadership they have integrated dimensions which are usually either explored separately or woefully neglected. We have long since left the hierarchical approach of "under supervision" to the approach of maximizing individual autonomy and group contribution by using our mentoring talents.

I believe that in our future, leaders will need to address profound issues that will test their knowledge, experience, and leadership competences. It is very necessary to introduce macroeconomics, consumerism, and marketing as essential to achieve skillful fiscal management. Clinicians must become savvy to the economic underpinnings of our service delivery as health care resources become scarcer and more competitive to obtain.

Quality assurance must not be left to languish or to become repetitive and potentially boring. The challenge to practitioners is to improve as individuals and team members; that will require continuous nurturing. The application of the concept of "Magnet Status" to the industry will create enthusiasm and pride. It will reap many benefits for the staff and institution and stimulate the achievement of continuous organizational health.

Cultural diversity is a clear indication of our changing society and must be incorporated into the philosophy of the institution. It is paramount that it be adopted and practiced by all personnel. The tools needed are education, team building, conflict management, and encouragement to understand and serve all the humanistic needs of our rapidly changing population.

The chaos of our health care system has created workplace stress. To diffuse this ongoing problem, leaders need applicable coping strategies. This can no longer be left to the human resources department alone. Because stress is evident in our daily workload and has a negative impact on productivity, leaders will need to be able to offer assistance and guidance at the worksite through creative workload assignments and staffing patterns.

The architecture of this book caught my attention and I believe that the authors worked together to develop an intriguing design to take the reader from theory to practice/application and into example. The reader will therefore be an active participant continuously interacting with the content of the text.

The insertion of the word 'renaissance' in the title signals by definition, "a new birth or revival" for transformational leadership. It emphasizes the fostering of a concept that has been very effective and productive as health professionals become more active participants in all aspects of health care delivery.

To break new ground—to stimulate ideas—to advance a body of knowledge—this is the challenge and hallmark of a meaningful instructional experience. It is what ensures the relevance and vitality of our professions. It is what is to be found within the covers of this book.

An advantage of writing the foreword to a text is to be among the first to view its content and design. My impression can best be summarized with a quotation from Victor Hugo, "Nothing in this world is as powerful as an idea whose time has come."

Samuel B. Feitelberg, PT, MA, FAPTA
Professor Emeritus, University of Vermont, 1997
Founding Dean, Center for Health Sciences
Clarkson University, 2005

Foreword

Laura Caramanica

The role of leadership in organizing and delivering high quality health care continues to grow in importance. Creating an environment that encourages and values the engagement of everyone in the institution is a key attribute of high-performing health care organizations, and a hallmark of Magnet hospitals. In Magnet hospitals, known for their ability to attract nurses and deliver excellent care, nursing and other leaders of patient care services use a participative management style, are highly visible, and communicate a compelling vision that inspires passion for making that vision a reality.

The definition of competencies for clinical managers is prerequisite for effective leadership across health care settings and professional disciplines, as is identification of theories and research that provide frameworks for analysis and decision making. Through presentation of the integrated multidimensional leadership model and excellent examples on how clinical managers can successfully foster horizontal and vertical communication, this new book is a must read for those who want to successfully combine the art and science of transformational leadership.

The authors have effectively selected and balanced theoretical and practical information that, along with the core competencies, enable clinical leaders to sustain excellence for themselves and for their organizations. This text should be of value for both graduate students and practicing clinical leaders as they continuously learn and improve their performance as leaders in the ever challenging health care arena.

Laura Caramanica, RN, PhD
Vice President for Nursing
Hartford Hospital
Hartford, Connecticut
Magnet Hospital, designated January 2002
Board of Directors, Region I
American Organization of Nurse Executives

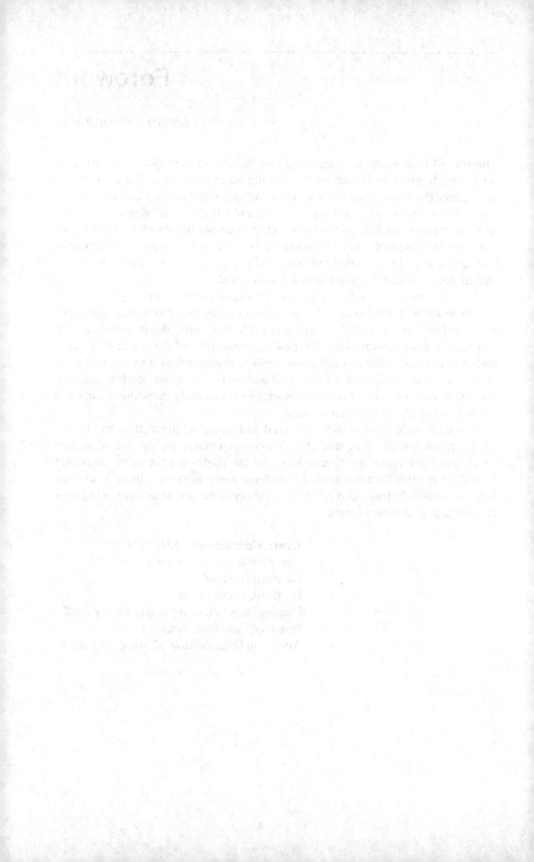

Introduction

WHO IS THIS BOOK FOR?

This book has been written for practicing clinical managers (nurses, physical therapists, occupational therapists, and so forth) and students in corresponding graduate programs. Today's practice environment encompasses a wide scope of clinical (versus discipline specific) leadership, where the focus is on patient care delivered by a multidisciplinary health care team. Although we have used a conversational tone geared specifically for practicing clinical managers, the book is peppered with theory applied to practice that graduate students require. The book is easily adapted for the academic environment and provides a foundation for supplemental readings in the scholarly literature.

WHAT APPROACH DOES THE BOOK TAKE?

Although the language of leadership varies, the basic principles of transformational leadership permeate the current organizational literature, including such strategies as visioning, building organizational trust, having self-confidence, and managing the organization to bring out the best in others. The adoption of these strategies by practicing clinical managers and leaders has been inconsistent, because of changes in the external environment in the last decade that have claimed the time and efforts of health care managers. In their landmark report, the Institute of Medicine (2003, p. 108) identified transformational leadership as one of the key strategies for transforming the work environment of nurses.

Transformational leadership alone is not enough. The real-world challenge for a leader is to figure out what knowledge or theory applies in each situation faced. We have tried to address this challenge in this book. In doing so, we develop and use a multidimensional model that includes:

- Transformational leadership, which provides both a theoretical and philosophical approach.

- Leadership IQ as presented by E. C. Murphy, which provides a more prescriptive approach to the development of leadership skills, consistent with transformational leadership.
- Leadership development through mentorship and professional development planning.
- Roles and competencies for clinical managers derived from a white paper published by VHA, Inc.

Each of these four approaches has been discussed separately elsewhere and in isolation of each other. In this book we integrate leadership skills into a role competency framework. Of course, simply reading a book will not increase a reader's leadership skills and role competencies. Thus, we ask the audience to actively read the book, engage in self-assessment, and develop a plan for leadership development, working with a mentor.

HOW IS THE BOOK ORGANIZED?

The book is divided into three parts. Part One introduces each of the elements of our multidimensional leadership model. Besides these four elements, we believe complexity science informs leadership practice, and it is presented in Chapter 5. Part One concludes with a chapter on managing personal resources because in order to be an effective leader you must lead a balanced life. Although more theoretical in approach than Part Two, these chapters are written in a conversational, easy-to-read style. Throughout the chapters there are self-assessment exercises, and each chapter ends with application exercises to assist the reader in applying theory to practice. We suggest that you read these chapters before reading Part Two, as they provide a foundation for how to practice leadership.

In Part Two we present seven role competencies:

- Customer needs and expectations
- Strategic visioning and strategic planning
- Managing care across the continuum
- Improving quality and performance
- Human resource management
- Marketing initiatives
- Financial outcomes

Starting with Chapter 8, at the conclusion of each chapter in Part Two, a real-life scenario is presented. The scenario shows how one of the more important aspects of the role competencies is applied in a practice setting. The scenario is then analyzed using transformational leadership, Leadership IQ, and complexity science as a framework, providing a link between Parts One and Two.

Part Three presents two real-life stories of leadership in practice. Chapter 16 describes how nurse leaders of Middlesex Hospital in Middletown, Connecticut, achieved Magnet status for their hospital. Clearly, the leadership to make this happen demonstrates transformational leadership at its best. The concluding chapter, "Complexity Science in Action," is a visionary and exciting story of Hunterdon Medical Center in Flemington, New Jersey and the willingness of its leaders to take risk and embrace this new science to manage and lead their organization. Linda Rusch, Vice President Patient Care Services, gives a profound account of their journey.

We have purposely not sought consistency in some terminology. We use the terms *patient, client,* and *customer* interchangeably. Further, we use both *clinical unit leader* and *clinical unit manager,* as your role is both leader and manager.

HOW CAN YOU APPLY THIS BOOK TO YOUR PRACTICE?

As you read, consider your organization's culture and how the organization has structured your role and set expectations. You can modify approaches and adopt strategies based on your assessment. Whether readers of this book work in large organizations that are highly bureaucratic or small entrepreneurial settings, we predict that the approaches we have suggested will work when you apply them in your own workplace.

As we undertook the journey of writing this book, one unexpected theme kept recurring: the whole is more than the sum of its parts. This book suggests a gestalt of leadership. Although you can apply one strategy or tool to your practice, only when you take most of what we suggest, reflect on it, and act, will you achieve a high-performance work team that works together to ensure positive client outcomes.

We salute both practicing and aspiring clinical managers who are at the front line of care delivery. You are in a position to influence the direction of health care in our nation. Happy reading!

Part One

CHAPTER 1

Leadership Practice: State of the Art and Recommendations for the Future

Anne M. Barker

────── **CHAPTER QUESTIONS** ──────

1. What is the current climate for leadership in health care organizations, and where should we be headed?
2. How can the development of transformational leadership theory over the last decade inform my current practice?
3. What are microsystems, and how can they help me see my role in a new way?
4. What are the four components of the leadership model that I can use to make me a more successful clinical manager?

INTRODUCTION

In this chapter we look at the practices and strategies of leadership over the last decade. It is our belief that during the 1990s the regulations of third parties and the almost desperate need to keep health care institutions financially viable took priority over concerns of leadership. However, we now recognize once again that human resources, the right ones, are the organization's strongest and most important assets. This introductory chapter provides a summary of leadership theory and suggests a model for implementing theory into practice for the future.

TRANSFORMATIONAL LEADERSHIP: TODAY'S REALITIES VERSUS YESTERDAY'S PREDICTIONS

In 1978 James McGregor Burns wrote a seminal book on leadership in which he coined the term *transformational leadership*. This theory differed from past theories in that it focused on meeting the needs and values of followers to motivate high performance in order to assure organizational success and goal at-

3

tainment. In the 1980s and into the 1990s this leadership theory and related strategies gained popularity in the business and health care industries. However, due to the financial constraints of the 1990s in health care organizations, leadership took a back seat as worries of organizational financial viability led to acquisitions and mergers, development of large integrated health care systems, job redesign, layoffs, mandatory reassignments of staff, and the closing of units and programs.

We believe that transformational leadership remains a viable, needed framework for managing in today's complex and chaotic health care environment. This belief is supported by the Institute of Medicine (2003, p. 108) who calls for transformational leadership as the strategy to keep patients safe. They support this call to action with research evidence. Although the language of leadership varies, the basic principles of transformational leadership permeate the current organizational literature, including such strategies as visioning, building organizational trust, having self-confidence, and managing the organization to bring out the best in others. We have observed that the adoption of these strategies by practicing clinical leaders has been inconsistent.

As we begin the new century, faced with a shortage of health care workers and a renewed recognition that human resources and their intellectual capital are the most important asset of the organization, we believe it is time to revisit and revitalize transformational leadership theory. *We do this in a framework of developing the competency and skills of clinical managers so that they can thrive in complex systems, where there are positive clinical outcomes for patients and a satisfying work environment for staff, achieved within the financial constraints of the system.*

In the next sections we look at some major concepts of transformational leadership, we review how these concepts developed over the last decade and propose how leadership should be developed in the future. These concepts include visioning, trust, self-esteem, and managing the organization.

Vision

The first major strategy of transformational leaders is to provide a vision of a possible and desirable future for the organization. In 1985 in their groundbreaking study of transformational leadership, Bennis and Nanus (p. 89) proposed that the vision must be realistic, attainable, credible, and attractive. Since that time visioning, vision statements, and value statements in health care organizations have gained wide popularity and use. Most—if not all—organizations have a vision and/or value statement.

We have two concerns about visions in many health care organizations. First, we are concerned that the visions for the whole organizational enterprise are superficial and are not guiding the actions and decisions of the organization. We believe that visions need to progress beyond written statements and slogans to be a set of values and beliefs that are lived. Wheatley (1992, p. 13) proposed that visions are "a force of unseen connections that influences employee behavior," and thus the next leadership challenge is to assure that the leaders in the organization internalize the vision and organizational values so that all decisions and actions in the organization, big and small, are measured against and are consistent with the vision. Further, leadership consistent with the organizational vision statement and values contributes significantly to the credibility of that leader within the institution.

The second concern we have about visions is that the individual units in the organization should have their own vision statements. Like that of the overall organization, the vision statements should guide the specific staff and patient population of that unit and be meaningful, living documents. In Chapter 9 we provide you with techniques to develop a vision for your unit, communicate it, and make it meaningful.

Organizational Trust

Organizational trust, the second transformational leadership strategy discussed here, is the foundation for developing positive, productive relationships between and among the clinical leader and staff (Bennis & Nanus, 1985). Trust is a complex sociological and psychological phenomenon, having many definitions.

In her 1992 work, Barker (p. 137) proposed that "the beliefs and behaviors of the leader-manager are the single most important determining factor of the development of organizational trust." However, in the 1990s, with organizational redesign leading to an overall feeling that staff are dispensable, employees became suspicious of managerial intent and motives and generally organizational trust deteriorated. The vestiges of these times remain today.

Building organizational trust is a complex yet essential strategy for health care organizational success for this century. Since trust begets trust and since trust starts with the leader, clinical leaders must recognize the importance of trust, assess trust levels, and design structures and processes for building trust in their setting. Moreover, we propose that future initiatives must not only be directed at building trust between the leader and followers but also must be directed to building trust among the entire team: trust must permeate the organization building a culture characterized by commitment to the customer, the team, and the organization's vision. In the next chapter we propose a model that describes leadership strategies to build and sustain organizational trust.

Self-Esteem

The third transformational leadership concept is self-esteem. Bennis and Nanus (1985) suggest that effective leaders must have high regard for themselves, not self-aggrandizement, but rather confidence in their role as manager. Their research on transformational leaders found that these leaders have high self-esteem and confidence in their role. What is important is that the leader's self-esteem results in their forming positive relationships with followers. Without high regard for oneself it is difficult, if not impossible, to have high regard for others. This book has been structured to help you develop leadership strategies and role competencies to enhance your self-esteem.

But the issues of self-esteem are greater than those of the leader. For the next decade, strategies to build staff self-esteem should be implemented. Staff must have confidence in their own roles and performance, receive positive feedback, and learn and grow in their roles.

Beyond self-esteem and for the future, the clinical leader and the staff must also find meaning and purpose in their work, referred to as self-actualization. By having a lived vision in which the staff shares values and beliefs and by having a work environment that allows the staff to achieve the vision, self-actualization needs can be met.

Managing the Organizational Structure: The Semiautonomous Work Unit to Microsystems

In the 1980s many authors argued that organizations would become a network of semiautonomous work units. For nursing, Barker (1992) suggested that each patient care unit would have its unique vision and goals, be given the freedom to make decisions for the unit, be further decentralized, and have shared power among the work group. She further predicted that the relationship with the central organization would be mutual versus authoritative.

At this time this vision for organizational structures has not been attained. The reasons for this are many: (1) the continued financial pressures for organizations to remain viable; (2) the rules and regulations governing health care organizations from the federal government, the state, accreditation agencies, and payers; and (3) the lack of experiences and models for designing these structures in health care organizations.

We believe the principles of semiautonomous work units should not be abandoned. Baker (2002) proposed that the needed changes in health care organizations will emerge from the redesign of patient care systems on the frontline versus reorganization of the larger systems. Certainly, the experiences of the last decade illustrate this. The mergers, acquisitions, and development of health care systems have not resulted in dramatic changes at the clinical unit level.

We believe that attention must be paid to clinical microsystems that are "small, functional, frontline units that provide most health care to most people. They are the essential building blocks of larger organizations and of the health system. They are the place where patients and providers meet. The quality and value of care produced by a large health system can be no better than the services generated by the small systems of which it is composed" (Nelson et al., 2002, p. 473).

In this book we focus on your role as the clinical manager of a microsystem. In health care this can be inpatient units, free-standing or inpatient clinics or departments, emergency departments, provider offices, home care units, and so forth. In the next chapter we discuss microsystems in more depth.

THE FUTURE: WHERE DO WE NEED TO GO?

The need for well-prepared clinical leaders to lead the changes in health care that promote cost-effective, quality health care outcomes for patients, families, and communities has been widely cited (American Hospital Association, 2002). While good quantitative data about the supply and demand for health care leaders is sparse, there is growing consensus and concern that there is a shortage of people choosing a career in management because of the pressures and frustrations placed on health care managers in today's complex health care environment. The dissatisfaction arises from a myriad of issues including financial constraints from payers, customer expectations, external rules and regulations, legal mandates, technological advances, and manpower shortages, to name a few. Moreover, the managerial workforce is aging and succession planning has been minimal.

Making the issue even more complex is the changing role of the clinical leader. The role is more demanding and has more responsibilities than a decade ago. New responsibilities and challenges are added constantly. Working collaboratively with multiple disciplines, and in some cases supervising members of other disciplines, calls for new skills and competencies. This book can assist you in developing these new skills, as you reflect on your role and your skills and knowledge.

THE LEADERSHIP MODEL

This book is organized using a model consisting of four concepts: (1) transformational leadership, (2) Leadership IQ, (3) clinical leadership role competencies, and (4) leadership development through mentorship and structured

Figure 1.1 Multidimensional Model of Leadership

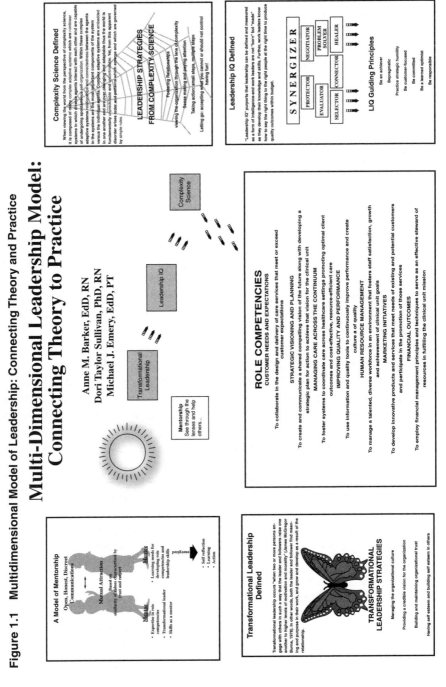

Multi-Dimensional Leadership Model:
Connecting Theory to Practice

Anne M. Barker, EdD, RN
Dori Taylor Sullivan, PhD, RN
Michael J. Emery, EdD, PT

Complexity Science Defined

When viewing the world from the perspective of complexity science, it is composed of many complex adaptive systems which are nonlinear systems in which diverse agents interact with each other and are capable of undergoing spontaneous self-organization. Within these complex adaptive systems, relationships and connections between the agents in the systems are the most significant components of the system versus the individual agents. Complex adaptive systems are embedded in one another and are ever-changing and adaptable thus the world is fundamentally unpredictable and unforeseeable. Yet, from this apparent disorder arises faster and patterned which emerge and which are governed by simple rules.

LEADERSHIP STRATEGIES FROM COMPLEXITY SCIENCE

Fostering Relationships
viewing the organization through the lens of complexity

Sense making and paying attention

Taking action/small steps, multiple steps

Letting go: accepting what you cannot or should not control
having fun!

Leadership IQ Defined

"Leadership IQ" purports that leadership can be defined and measured as a form of intelligence and work leaders are not "born" but "made" as they develop their knowledge and skills. Further, work leaders know how to say the right thing to the right people at the right time to produce quality outcomes within budget.

S Y N E R G I Z E R

PROTECTOR — NEGOTIATOR
EVALUATOR — PROBLEM SOLVER
SELECTOR — CONNECTOR — HEALER

LIQ Guiding Principles

Be an achiever
Be pragmatic
Practice strategic humility
Be customer-focused
Be committed
Be a learned optimist
Be responsible

ROLE COMPETENCIES
CUSTOMER NEEDS AND EXPECTATIONS

To collaborate in the design and delivery of care services that meet or exceed customer expectations

STRATEGIC VISIONING AND PLANNING

To create and communicate a shared compelling vision of the future along with developing a strategic plan for action to achieve that vision for the clinical unit

MANAGING CARE ACROSS THE CONTINUUM

To foster systems to coordinate care across healthcare settings promoting optimal client outcomes and cost-effective, resource-efficient care

IMPROVING QUALITY AND PERFORMANCE

To use information and quality tools to continuously improve performance and create culture a of quality

HUMAN RESOURCE MANAGEMENT

To manage a talented, diverse workforce in an environment that fosters staff satisfaction, growth and achievement of clinical unit goals

MARKETING INITIATIVES

To develop innovative products and services that meet needs of existing and potential customers and participate in the promotion of those services

FINANCIAL OUTCOMES

To employ financial management principles and techniques to serve as an effective steward of resources in fulfilling the clinical unit mission

Complexity Science

Leadership IQ

Transformational Leadership

Mentorship
See through the lenses and help others....

A Model of Mentorship

Open, Honest, Discreet Communications

Mutual Attraction
Based on similarity of values characterized by trust and respect

Mentor
• Expertise in role competencies
• Transformational leader
• Skills as a mentor

Mentee
• Learning needs for developing role competencies and leadership skills

Mentoring

• Self reflection
• Learning
• Action

Transformational Leadership Defined

Transformational leadership occurs "when two or more persons engage with others in such a way that the leader and followers raise one another to higher levels of motivation and morality" (James McGregor Burns, 1978). In other words, both the leader and follower find meaning and purpose in their work, and grow and develop as a result of the relationship.

TRANSFORMATIONAL LEADERSHIP STRATEGIES

Managing the organizational culture

Providing a credible vision for the organization

Building and maintaining organizational trust

Having self esteem and building self esteem in others

learning. Figure 1.1 is an illustration of the model. Each concept is discussed below with in-depth information in the following chapters. Additionally, the environment in which you practice is a complex system and the implications of that are covered in Chapter 5.

Transformational Leadership

The theory of transformational leadership underpins the model and is discussed in detail in Chapter 2. This theory complements and works well when using complexity science to understand organizations (Chapter 5).

In practice, transformational leadership is a philosophical point of view about the leader-follower relationship versus a prescriptive set of rules and guidelines. The leader-follower relationship is an engagement of both parties for the shared benefit of the organization, the people it serves, and the people who work in the organization. This view provides the framework for how leaders think about themselves, about leading others, and about followers.

Transformational leaders have an optimistic worldview that focuses on the positive and possibilities. Further, they understand that leadership is ethical and that leaders have a fiduciary responsibility in which they must place the concerns of others over their own. By virtue of being in a formal leadership position, clinical managers have special knowledge, authority, and power, and have a moral obligation not to abuse it. This lays a foundation for developing trusting relationships.

Leadership IQ

Leadership IQ, which complements both transformational leadership theory and role competencies, provides the second concept to the model and is discussed in detail in Chapter 3. This concept has been developed by Murphy (1996) from research spanning 20 years and observation of and/or surveys of over 1,000 managers. In summary, Murphy (1996, pp. 5–6) found that successful leaders know "how to say the right thing to the right people at the right time to get the right work done well, on time and within budget." Chapter 3 examines each of the specific roles and tools used but in summary leaders demonstrating the principles of Leadership IQ know how to:

- Select the right people.
- Connect them to the right cause.
- Solve problems that arise.
- Evaluate progression toward objectives.

- Negotiate resolutions to conflicts.
- Heal the wounds inflicted by change.
- Protect their cultures from the perils of crisis.
- Synergize all stakeholders in a way that enables them to achieve improvements together (Murphy, 1996, p. 4).

Leadership Role Competencies

Although these values and beliefs of transformational leadership are essential for success, they are not enough and cannot stand alone. The clinical leader needs the knowledge and skills to be competent in his or her role and to use these in a manner consistent with transformational leadership. The role competencies in the model have been adapted from the VHA, Inc. (2000) white paper on the role of the chief nursing officer. Although these competencies were originally categorized and identified for the chief nursing officer, they are a comprehensive and useful framework for all clinical managers at any level of the organization. The focus and necessity for the competency might vary from role to role at different levels in the organization, but the competencies are an appropriate way to categorize the knowledge and skills needed to be an effective clinical leader in health care today. In the model there are seven competencies. The chapters in Part Two of this book address these competencies:

- Identifying and meeting customer needs and expectations
- Participating in the development and implementation of the organizational vision and strategic plan
- Developing and managing clinical care delivery systems
- Promoting quality improvement and building a culture of quality by managing information to monitor and measure the quality, safety, and appropriateness of care and services
- Leading others in the workforce to provide clinically competent care
- Marketing clinical services
- Managing financial resources effectively and efficiently

Professional Development and Mentorship

The fourth component of the model is professional development and mentoring. To become an effective clinical leader takes a thoughtful, planned journey of self-assessment, reflection, and goal setting. In this model professional development is two-pronged: working with a mentor and setting goals and evaluating progress toward goal completion.

Although there are many definitions of a mentor, for this book we have adopted the classic definition proposed by Vance (1982). She defines a mentor as an experienced person who guides and nurtures a less experienced person (the mentee). The mentor is someone who inspires, instructs, nurtures, and encourages the mentee. Vance states that the mentoring relationship is a helping relationship that is special, emotional, intense, and enduring as opposed to shorter term and less intense relationships such as preceptor, sponsor, role model, or peer.

In Chapter 4 we present our model of mentorship in which the relationship between the mentor and mentee can best be described as a partnership. In entering into this partnership, there is a congruency between the expertise and the organizational connections of the mentor and the learning needs of the mentee. As a result of the relationship and interactions between the two, the mentee is energized for self-reflection, learning, and action, leading to professional role development and growth.

A mentor-mentee relationship may develop from close associations and working relationships or through formal mentorship programs. Any readers who do not have a mentor should seek out someone to guide and support them through their professional development and use of this book. Chapter 4 discusses the roles of the mentee and the mentor and their relationship to assist you in identifying a mentor and in setting up a working relationship.

Along with a mentor, clinical leaders need to have a systematic goal-oriented approach for professional development. One unique characteristic of this book is that many chapters have one or more self- and/or organizational assessments, and every chapter has application exercises designed to enhance your leadership skills. The application exercises can help you apply what you have read and put it into practice.

APPLICATION EXERCISES

Complete the following exercises as preparation for reading the rest of the book.

1. Briefly reflect on your organization's vision, the level of organizational trust, and your own feelings of self-esteem.
2. Review the leadership IQ roles and reflect on which you believe to be your greatest strengths and weaknesses.
3. Review the seven leadership competencies and reflect on which you believe to be your greatest strengths and weaknesses.

REFERENCES

American Hospital Association (2002). *In our hands: How hospital leaders can build a thriving workforce.* Retrieved May 16, 2002, from http://hospitalconnect.com.

Baker, G. R. (2002). Healthcare managers in the complex world of healthcare. *Frontiers of Health Service Management, 18* (2), 23–32.

Barker, A. M. (1992). *Transformational nursing leadership: A vision for the future.* New York: National League for Nursing Press.

Bennis, W., & Nanus, B. (1985). *Leaders: The strategies for taking charge.* New York: Harper & Row.

Burns, J. M. (1978). *Leadership.* New York: Harper & Row.

Institute of Medicine. (2003). Keeping patients safe: Transforming the work environment of nurses. Washington, DC: Author.

Murphy, E. C. (1996). *Leadership IQ: A personal development process based on a scientific study of a new generation of leaders.* New York: John Wiley & Sons.

Nelson, E. C., Batalden, P. B., Huber, T. P., Mohr, J. J., Godfrey, M. M., Headrick, J. H., et al. (2002). Microsystems in health care: Part 1. Learning from high performing front-line clinical units. *Joint Commission Journal on Quality and Safety, 29,* 472–497.

Vance, C. (1982). The mentor connection. *Journal of Nursing Administration, 12* (4), 7–13.

VHA, Inc. (2000). *Revolutionizing the future of nursing care: Defining the role of the chief nursing officer in the 21st century.* [Brochure]. Dallas: Author.

Wheatley, M. J. (1992). *Leadership and the new science: Learning about organization from an orderly universe.* San Francisco: Berrett-Koehler Publishers.

CHAPTER 2

Transformational Leadership Practice: Designing High-Performing Clinical Units

Anne M. Barker

--------- **CHAPTER QUESTIONS** ---------

1. What is transformational leadership and how can I practice it?
2. What are the characteristics of a high-performing clinical unit?
3. What is organizational trust and why is it important?
4. What strategies can I use to increase trust in my unit?
5. What techniques can I use to increase the self-esteem of the staff?
6. What is organizational culture and how can I assess it?

INTRODUCTION

In this chapter we focus on current and future practices to develop your skills as a transformational leader. We discuss three of the four transformational leadership strategies first introduced in Chapter 1: the organizational structure, organizational trust, and self-esteem. Since an entire chapter is devoted to visioning and strategic planning, we will consider the development and communication of organizational visions later.

LEADERSHIP SELF-AWARENESS

Starting in this chapter, you will begin to assess and reflect on your leadership and management strengths and weaknesses in order to develop a plan to enhance your skills and reach your career goals. In many of the chapters that follow, there will be an assessment for you to reflect on your leadership skills and competencies. In Chapter 4 we discuss selecting and working with a mentor to help you develop your leadership skills further.

13

One of the dilemmas and realities of reading a book is that you are not going to improve your leadership by just reading the book. You have to embrace what you find useful and what resonates for you. We hope your goal in reading this book is to increase your self-awareness, meaning having a deep understanding of your emotions, as well as your strengths and limitations (Goleman, Boyatzis, & McKee, 2002).

Table 2.1 is a leadership self-assessment for you to take to increase your self-awareness. This assessment focuses on the skills and strategies needed for transformational leadership. Taking this assessment before reading the chapter can help you focus on those aspects where you feel you need the most information and support. At the conclusion of the chapter, you can then develop one or more goals for yourself based on the assessment and the knowledge you gained from reading this chapter.

Table 2.1   Leadership Self-Assessment

This exercise is designed to help you think about your leadership skills and increase your self-awareness.

Transformational Leadership Strategies

- What are your values and beliefs about client care, your profession, and health care that can help you articulate a vision?
- In three to five sentences write down your vision. Is it intellectually stimulating? Credible? Easy to understand?
- How do you think people view your trustworthiness and integrity?
- Does your behavior align with your words and your vision?
- Are you able to stay positive, optimistic, and passionate about your work?
- Do you provide coaching, support, and positive feedback to the staff frequently? How do you think your staff would rate your ability to do this?
- How confident are you in your role?
  - What experiences do you have to build on?
  - What new experiences do you need to move into the future?
  - What knowledge do you have to build on?
  - What new knowledge do you need to move into the future?
  - What are your strengths?
  - What are your limitations?

Career Goals

- What are your career goals? What is stopping you? What are you doing about it?
- What networks do you have in place to help you?
- What new relationships do you need to develop to help you?

TRANSFORMATIONAL LEADERSHIP: THEORETICAL BACKGROUND

Ancient scholars and philosophers such as Plato and Confucius observed, wrote about, and analyzed leadership, but it was not until the 1930s and the onset of World War II that one can find formal theories and empirical studies of leadership. Until the emergence of the theory of transformational leadership in 1978, leadership theories and studies focused on the role of the manager and the manager's relationship with followers.

During these four decades, several important themes emerged that still have relevance in today's organizations. First, most theories purported that the democratic participatory style with positive supportive relationships between the manager and the follower is generally more effective than autocratic styles of leadership (White & Lippit, 1960; Fielder, 1967; Likert, 1967). Second, the leader must pay attention to organizational goals (House, 1971; Blake & Mouton, 1985). And last, the theories purported, and research studies further supported, that the behaviors and attitudes of the leader affect follower satisfaction and group performance (White & Lippit, 1960; Fielder, 1967).

Barker (1992, p. 14) argued that these theories are not wrong, but are simply unfinished and do not help explain what makes organizations successful and the people working in the organization enthusiastic. Further, they do not consider in enough depth the values and motives that workers bring to their work.

To address this deficit, in 1978 James McGregor Burns identified a new leadership theory that he called transformational leadership. In his seminal work, *Leadership*, Burns, a social scientist, described the leadership style and strategies of famous political leaders such as Mahatma Gandhi, Franklin Roosevelt, and John Kennedy. This work has resonated with organizational scholars and practitioners and forms the basis for most of the contemporary writing about leadership. During the 1980s and continuing today, there's been a major paradigm shift in our view of leadership from a focus on tasks and systems of controls to one of building the organizational culture to provide an environment in which people are successful and organizational outcomes are positive.

Burns (1978, p. 18) defined the leadership situation as occurring when "persons with certain motives and purposes mobilize, in competition or conflict with others, institutional, political, psychological, and other resources to arouse, engage and satisfy the motives of followers." Looking at this definition, essential to leadership is a leader with motives and purposes that are positive and productive and followers whose needs are met and satisfied. Further, leadership generally occurs in situations where there are conflicting purposes and competition.

Burns (1978, p. 20) goes on to define *transformational leadership* as occurring "when two or more persons engage with others in such a way that the leader and followers raise one another to higher levels of motivation and morality." In other words, both the leader and follower find meaning and purpose in their work, and grow and develop as a result of the relationship.

In contrast to transformational leadership, Burns (1978) describes a form of leadership called *transactional leadership*. He defines this as the leader taking the initiative to make contact with others for the purpose of an exchange. In organizations this exchange is salary and recognition for service. It is thought to be the more common form of leadership and seen more often than transformational leadership. In the exchange that occurs in a transactional situation, the needs of both the leader and the follower are met; however, their purposes are separate and not related. They are not bound together in pursuit of a common vision or direction.

In the definition of transformational leadership, it is important to emphasize that the role of the transformational leader is to satisfy the needs of followers and thus motivate them to high levels of performance. Burns' focus is on higher level needs such as self-esteem and self-actualization. His work relied heavily on Maslow's hierarchy of needs.

According to Maslow (1970), human beings have six categories of needs: physiological, safety, belongingness and love, self-esteem, self-actualization, and aesthetics. These needs are arranged in a hierarchy beginning with physiological needs and ending with aesthetics needs. In other words, generally one set of needs does not arise until the more basic needs are fulfilled. As an example, humans are not as concerned for their security and safety (the second level of human needs) until the physiological needs for food, water, and sleep are met. Typically, in health care organizations most attention has been paid to the first three levels of needs. Efforts have been in place to pay salaries that afford people their basic physiological needs, to provide a safe working environment, and to have a sense of belonging to the organization through such efforts as shared governance and participatory management.

For the future, it is important that attention be paid to the self-esteem and self-actualization needs of employees. We discuss this more later in this chapter. Transformational leaders motivate followers to move beyond their self-interest and to contribute to the overall vision and success of the organization. By doing so, the followers then meet their need for finding meaning and purpose in their work and may, according to Burns (1978), become leaders themselves.

Although the major focus of his work was on well-known political leaders, Burns (1978) argued that transformational leadership can be found in all aspects of daily life such as in parents, teachers, and business leaders. And indeed, based on his work, many organizational scholars have studied and written about transformational leadership, most notably Bennis and Nanus (1985), Bennis (2003), and Bass and Avolio (1993).

Bennis and Nanus (1985) provided one of the first landmark studies of transformational leadership. In observing over 90 CEOs of Fortune 500 companies, they found four important leadership strategies. Furthering this work and in an effort to develop an instrument to measure transformational leadership, Bass and Avolio (1993) described similar characteristics but used different terminology. Consolidating the work of these authors, the following transformational leadership strategies are identified and discussed in our model:

- *Managing the organizational culture of the organization through intellectual stimulation of the follower.* Transformational leaders provide a learning environment by encouraging questioning, challenging assumptions, asking people to think out-of-the-box, and fostering creativity and innovation.
- *Providing a credible vision for the organization and inspiring others.* Transformational leaders motivate and inspire followers by providing a vision, designing meaningful work environments to achieve the vision, building self-esteem, and staying optimistic and enthusiastic.
- *Building and maintaining organizational trust so that the leader can influence follower performance.* Transformational leaders behave in such a way that they are trusted, admired, and respected.
- *Having self-esteem and building self-esteem in others, so that individual consideration is given to each follower.* Transformational leaders engage with followers and treat each person as unique; emphasize growth and development; and support, coach, and mentor the staff.

DEVELOPING TRANSFORMATIONAL LEADERSHIP SKILLS

In this section we look at three of the four transformational leadership strategies in greater depth. First, we look at structuring the clinical unit consistent with leadership strategies that promote a successful and enthusiastic workplace. We then look closely at the issues of organizational trust and self-esteem.

Managing the Organizational Structure: High-Performing Clinical Units

As we indicated previously, the focus of this book is on the clinical unit as a microsystem of a larger organization (macrosystem). To review, the following are the characteristics of a microsystem:

- They are small frontline units where the work of the organization happens.
- It is where the provider and the patient interact.

- The microsystem is responsible for the quality of care delivered and the value of that care.
- The larger system, or organization, is only as successful as the sum of all the microsystems.
- The staff in the microsystems are loyal first to their patients and then to the microsystem. There is rarely any loyalty to the overall organization (Mohr, Batalden, & Barach, 2004).

Table 2.2 lists characteristics of high-performance microsystems. It has been designed by synthesizing the work of Nelson et al. (2002) with our model of

---

Table 2.2   Characteristics of a High-Performance Clinical Unit

Clinical Unit (Microsystem)

- Complex adaptive systems
- Embedded in the organization (macrosystem)
- Embedded in the health care delivery system and society
- Organizational culture characterized by being mission driven, having concern for the quality of work life, demanding respectful team relationships, and promoting learning

Clinical Leader

- Transformational leader
- Uses strategies of Leadership IQ and role competencies
- Views the organizations through the lens of complexity

Staff

- Connected team of multidisciplinary staff
- Satisfied
- Loyal to the unit and patients
- High performance

Subpopulation of Patients

- Quality outcomes
- Patient satisfaction
- Cost effective

Processes

- Information
- Performance improvement
- System design

transformational leadership. In Chapter 5 we give more details about complexity science and complex adaptive systems for furthering your understanding of complexity science. For now, suffice it to say that your *clinical unit* is a complex system that is embedded in another complex system, the organization or macrosystem. The culture of this unit is characterized by being mission driven, having a concern for the quality of staff work life, supporting learning and growth, and having respectful patterns of staff interaction. The unit is led by a *transformational leader* who is competent in the many roles needed to lead the unit and who embraces the complexity of the work. The *staff* is a cohesive, connected team characterized by trust, collaboration, and respect. The primary focus of the team is on the patient. There are high expectations for staff to perform, to learn, and to network. The *patients* in the microsystem are a subpopulation of patients with specific health care needs and as a result of the interaction with the staff experience quality care, appreciate its value, and are satisfied with the clinical unit's care. Three organizational *processes* are needed to carry out the work of the microsystem. The first is information flow aided by information technology, performance improvement supported by continuous monitoring of care, and systems designed to provide quality, cost-effective, and efficient care.

We use this model as a framework throughout the book. As the leader of a microsystem, you must pay attention to all the components of the microsystem to build an organizational culture for high performance. As we repeat throughout the book, all these strategies are used in concert with one another and are synergistic.

Organizational Trust

The importance of organizational trust cannot be overstated. First and foremost, the clinical leader cannot actualize the strategies of transformational leadership unless she is trusted by followers. The leader's ability to appeal to the values of followers is directly related to whether she is trusted by them. Further, the work of the health care team involves a great deal of interdependence on each other. In fact, it would be hard to cite an example in which successful client care occurred due to the efforts of only one person. Trust is the foundation upon which leadership and team relationships can be built and flourish. The role of the clinical leader is to build an organizational culture characterized by trust.

Barker (1992) proposes that the single most important determining factor of organizational trust are the behaviors and values of the clinical leader. At its foundation trust begets trust, and distrust begets distrust. Thus, it is the responsibility of the leader to display trusting behaviors, to trust others, and to build organizational trust. If done correctly, followers will trust the leader. It is not inherent that followers trust their leader simply by virtue of their position in the organization. Rather, it is the leader that must start the cycle of trust. Trust must be earned and nurtured every day and in every situation. It takes time, patience, and unending attention.

In this section we first define trust and then consider the behaviors of the leader that create and sustain trust. We then discuss the positive effects on the functioning of the organization when trust exists.

Definition and Meaning of Trust

That there are no universally accepted definitions of trust is a reflection that trust is multidimensional having both psychological and sociological features, having both collective and individual aspects, and developing along a time dimension. Scholars who have written about trust vary in their definition of trust and how trust is developed, but many commonalities are also seen. We have attempted to consolidate the information in the literature so that it is easy for you to use in your practice.

Mayer and Davis (1996) define trust as "the willingness of a party to be vulnerable to the actions of another party based on the expectation that the other will perform a particular action important to the truster irrespective of the ability to monitor or control the other party." If you look closely at this definition, it may help you to understand how difficult developing trust can be. Trust means you must allow yourself to be vulnerable to another person and believe that person will act in a way that is beneficial to you.

Further, Zand (1972, p. 230) identified a phenomenon called the "short-cycle feedback loop." He identified that trust begets trust, and mistrust begets mistrust. According to Zand, trusting behaviors increase mutual trust. For example, a trusting clinical manager will be open and honest, communicate fully and accurately, and exert fewer rigid controls on others. This results in the follower trusting the leader and in turn communicating fully and working mutually with the leader, increasing the leader's trust in the follower with a cycle of trust developing. On the other hand, leaders who exhibit distrusting behaviors, withhold information, are not honest and open, and are controlling of others will not gain the trust of the followers. Followers will then withhold information, resist influence, and not work toward mutual goals, causing the manager to distrust them and a cycle of distrust develops.

Leadership Strategies That Promote Trust

In this section we suggest strategies you can adopt to develop organizational trust. Table 2.3 summarizes these strategies into five distinct dimensions: behavioral integrity, communications, character, competence, and influence and control.

Table 2.3   Leadership Behaviors That Promote Trust

Behavioral Integrity	Honesty and Moral Character
• Sincere	• Ethical behavior
• Consistent and dependable	• Good intentions
• Fulfills promises	**Competency and Credibility**
Communications	• Technical
	• Interpersonal
• Open	• Decision making
• Accurate	• Leadership effectiveness
• Honest	**Influence and Control**
• Timely	• Mutual goal setting
• Concern	• Empowerment

In our model the first strategy is *behavioral integrity*. In his review of the literature about trust, Simons (2002) noted that there is substantial agreement that one of the key antecedents for the development of trust is the perceived alignment of a person's deeds with his words. A common expression for this is "walking the talk." In our model this is the first dimension of trust. As a leader you must be sincere, fulfill promises that you make, and be consistent and dependable in what you do.

The next set of leadership strategies for the development of organizational trust involves *communications*. Communications has two elements—knowing what to communicate and when to communicate it. Communications need to be open, accurate, honest, and timely. This includes communications about the organization, such as new policies, issues, and future direction as well as sharing feelings and values. It also includes one-to-one communication with others; for example, giving constructive and honest feedback to employees about their performance. At the same time, the clinical leader needs to know when to keep information confidential and when to be discreet and not engage in gossip and harmful rumor spreading. In chapter 13 we further discuss communication competencies.

The third strategy is found in the *character of the leader* and includes characteristics such as displaying basic honesty and moral character, acting ethically and with good intentions and motives, and fulfilling one's fiduciary obligations. The clinical manager's fiduciary responsibility means placing the concern of others above one's own. Fiduciary responsibilities are moral obligations placed upon individuals with specialized knowledge, skill, and power. As a manager in the organization, the clinical leader has more resources, knowledge, and power than the staff, so these must be used for the benefit of clients and staff in the organization, not in one's own self-interest.

The next set of leadership strategies are those that are based in the *competence and credibility* of the leader. Clinical leaders must be technically competent in their profession, demonstrating an understanding of the clinical issues. Further, the leader must be competent in interpersonal skills in working with others and in their management and leadership skills. This leads to belief in the leader as a credible practitioner and manager, one that people want to follow. And lastly, the clinical leader needs to demonstrate good decision-making skills so that followers develop a trust in the decisions that are made and changes that occur. Followers often measure this dimension by whether the unit is well run with positive outcomes for the patients and the design of a satisfying work environment.

The last group of strategies for the development of organizational trust is in the area of *influence and control*. The way in which the leader and followers should influence one another is in setting mutual goals and directions together. Also, the leader exerts control over the organization through empowerment, versus power wielding. Empowerment is a process that includes giving the staff the opportunity to take action; providing them the resources to be successful, including time, money, space, and so forth; supporting their efforts; and providing the necessary information to get the work done (Kanter, 1993). As we will see in Chapter 5 on complexity science, organizations are essentially unpredictable and uncontrollable, and the most effective strategy for the leader is to help staff make connections that allow changes to emerge.

The Positive Influence of Organizational Trust

To repeat an earlier statement, the importance of organizational trust cannot be overstated. Throughout the literature on this topic the following positive organizational outcomes have been associated with high levels of organizational trust:

- Enhanced employee performance
- Improved organizational effectiveness
- Greater commitment to the organization
- Good communications and information sharing
- Less resistance to organizational change
- Improved team functioning

- Improved job satisfaction/retention
- Greater participation in decision making and problem solving

Self-Esteem

The most essential personal trait of successful transformational leaders is having a positive self-regard (Bennis & Nanus, 1985, p. 57). For our purposes, we use Maslow's (1970, pp. 45–46) classic definition of self-esteem. Maslow suggests that self-esteem is a stable, firmly based, high evaluation of self or self-respect. It includes important attributes such as the need for achievement, for developing competencies in one's role, for being confident, for feeling independent, and being able to act freely. When the self-esteem need is satisfied, the person feels self-confident, worthy, strong, capable, adequate, useful, and necessary.

Self-esteem is generated from authentic capacity, competency, and performance. It comes from what the person believes about himself or herself, not from the opinions of others. Self-esteem is not self-centeredness, cockiness, self-worship, or self-aggrandizement.

As part of your self-assessment, we offer three methods to develop a high self-regard. These are (1) completing the self-assessment exercises and using a mentor to recognize your strengths and weaknesses and develop a plan to compensate for weaknesses; (2) nurturing your talents and skills by goal setting and goal attainment; and (3) assessing the fit between your talents and skills and what the organization requires.

One other technique for increasing self-esteem is to have positive self-expectations. Expectations are extremely important yet subconscious determinants of behavior. How you see yourself and what you expect dictate how you act. A phenomenon called the *Wallenda factor* illustrates this point. Carl Wallenda, a successful tightrope artist, fell to his death as a result of focusing too much attention and worry about falling, sometimes referred to as "what you think about you bring about!" For some reason, he became obsessed about falling—and he did. His story has become a frequently cited example of how expectations drive behaviors.

It is beyond the scope of this book to suggest detailed methods for development of your own self-esteem. However, it is important that you take some time to reflect on how you feel about yourself as a clinical leader. Some thoughtful, honest self-reflection on the leadership assessment at the beginning of this chapter is a good place to begin. Further, getting feedback from your mentor and your boss can also provide you with valuable information for increasing your self-esteem. Two popular methods for assisting one to increase self-esteem are affirmation and visualization. There are good self-help books, tapes, and videos that you may wish to use.

Damage to Self-Esteem

One of the biggest detriments to one's self-esteem is the perceived need to be perfect and to avoid mistakes. Since no one is or can be perfect, this is an unrealistic standard against which to measure yourself. Perfectionists can never live up to their own expectations and often have a sense of failure, which in turn, lowers their self-esteem. Further, people striving for perfection may subconsciously avoid taking risks in order to avoid failure, leading to decreased role competence.

Another issue that can damage the self-esteem of health care professionals is all the bad press and publicity that health care receives today. For instance, the recent press about patient deaths due to medical errors can affect the way we think about the health care system in which we work and the profession in which we practice. As leaders, we need to counteract the negative issues with celebrating and appreciating the positive accomplishments and contributions that our staff make daily.

Developing Self-Esteem in Others

Besides attending to one's own self-esteem, the clinical leader has the responsibility to enhance the self-esteem of the people they supervise. Although not solely responsible for other people's self-esteem, the clinical manager plays an important role in either diminishing or enhancing the self-esteem of others, especially related to their work competency and mastery.

One of the most important techniques in the clinical leader's arsenal is setting realistic but high expectations for the staff, known as the self-filling prophecy, or the *Pygmalion effect*. The essence of the Pygmalion effect is that a person, by his will and effort, can transform another person through his expectation of another. The name came from the Greek sculptor Pygmalion, who sculpted a beautiful statue and then fell in love with her and willed her to come alive. And according to the mythology she did!

People live up to the subtle, at times unconscious, expectation of others, just as one lives up to one's own expectations for oneself. If the clinical leader sets high, realistic, and achievable expectations for employee performance and productivity, people will live up to them. On the other hand, when the leader has low or negative expectations of others, they will also live down to them. When expectations are low, people's self-esteem is not built.

The classic yet still pertinent research study by Livingston (1969) found evidence that supports the existence of this phenomenon in organizations. Livingston found that the expectations that the leader has of followers directly affects their organizational performance and career progress. Superior managers have a unique ability to be able to create high performance expectations for followers. This characteristic seems to emerge from managers' confidence in their own skill to develop others. On the other hand, less effective managers do not expect the same high level of performance; consequently, their people do not perform as well. Further, these managers have less confidence in their own abilities to set high expectations. In conclusion, staff most often behave in the way they think they are expected to behave.

Telling people when they are doing a good job (this tells the person what the expectation is) is seemingly simple advice, but the rationale for this is much more powerful than simply giving positive feedback—it is setting expectations and rewarding the positive outcomes.

A personal observation of the author is that high-performing health care teams are led by a leader who believes in the staff and frequently states that this is the best team in the organization! It is difficult to know for certain which comes first. But analyzing this through the theory of expectations, telling the staff that they are the best means they will become the best.

In summary, and most important, the clinical leader must make a conscious effort to focus on the positive. This includes giving positive and frequent feedback to individuals, as well as to the entire team. A simple technique to do this is to frequently and consciously seek out people doing the right thing and then provide them with positive feedback.

ORGANIZATIONAL CULTURE

It is important to appreciate that transformational leadership practice occurs within an organizational context and that each organization has its own culture that affects your practice. The study of organizational culture became popular in the 1980s. At that time Deal and Kennedy (1982) defined organizational culture as the values, beliefs, and behaviors that are shared by members of the organization. Furthering this definition in 1992, Schein proposed that organizational culture is a pattern of shared basic assumptions that a group learns as it solves problems. These assumptions used routinely and unconsciously are taught to new members of the organization as the correct way to do things.

Peters and Waterman devised a 7-S framework for assessing organizational culture. They proposed that seven components, when taken together, define an organization's culture:

- Style
- Structure
- Systems

Table 2.4   Organizational Culture Assessment

Style
- What are the management styles of the executive managers? Does any one style predominate?
- What is really important and valued?
- What five words describe your organization?

Structure
- Looking at the organizational chart, how would you describe the structure? Who reports to whom and why?
- How is the work divided? By functional area? Service line?

Systems
- What are the formal management systems (human resources, information, financial, etc.)?
- Which work well and which do not?

Skills
- What does the organization do well as compared to its competitors? What skills are missing?

Staff
- Who comprises the staff?
- What behaviors are rewarded? Who gets promoted?

Symbols
- What are the symbols that the organization uses?
- What are the ceremonies, rites, and rituals?
- Who are the heroes? What are the myths?

Shared Values
- What are the real shared values (these are not necessarily the written values!)?

- Skills
- Staff
- Symbols
- Shared values (Valuebasedmanagement.net, 2004)

In the framework of these seven components, Table 2.4 lists questions for determining the culture of your organization. Use this tool to assess the larger organization and the culture of your clinical unit.

APPLICATION EXERCISES

1. Using Table 2.1 and Table 2.3, write down three things you can do to increase your trustworthiness in the eyes of your staff.
2. Using Table 2.2, assess the strengths and weaknesses of your clinical unit.
3. Using Table 2.4, answer the questions to gain a better understanding of your organizational culture. What did you learn and how might this inform your leadership practice?

REFERENCES

Barker, A. M. (1992). *Transformational nursing leadership: A vision for the future*. New York: National League for Nursing.

Bass, B. M., & Avolio, B. J. (1993). *Improving organizational effectiveness through transformational leadership*. Thousand Oaks, CA: Sage.

Bennis, W. (2003). *On becoming a leader: The leadership classic—updated and expanded* (rev. ed.). New York: Perseus Publishing.

Bennis, W. B., & Nanus, B. (1985). *Leaders: The strategies for taking charge*. New York: John Wiley & Sons.

Blake, R. R., & Mouton, J. S. (1985). *The managerial grid III*. Houston: Gulf Publishing.

Burns, J. M. (1978). *Leadership*. New York: Harper & Row.

Deal, T. & Kennedy, A. (1982). *Corporate cultures: The rites and rituals of corporate life*. Reading, MA: Addison-Wesley Publishing Co.

Fielder, F. E. (1967). *A theory of leadership effectiveness*. New York: McGraw-Hill.

Goleman, D., Boyatzis, R., & McKee, A. (2002). *Primal leadership: Realizing the power of emotional intelligence*. Boston: Harvard Business School Press.

House, R. J. (1971). A path goal theory of leadership effectiveness. *Administrative Science Quarterly, 16*, 321–338.

Kanter, R. (1993). *Men and women of the corporation* (2nd ed.). New York: Basic Books.

Likert, R. (1967). *The human organization: Its management and values*. New York: McGraw-Hill.

Livingston, J. S. (1969). Pygmalion in management. *Harvard Business Review, 47*(3), 81–89.

Maslow, A. H. (1970). *Motivation and personality* (2nd ed.). New York: Harper & Row.

Mayer, R. C., & Davis, J. H. (1996). An integrative model of organizational trust. *Academic Management Review, 20*(3), 709–734.

McKinsey 7-S Framework model. Retrieved April 12, 2005, from http://www.valuebased management.net/methods_7S.html.

Mohr, J. J., Batalden, P., & Barach (2004). Integrating patient safety into the clinical microsystem. *Joint Commission Journal on Quality and Safety, 13*(Suppl II), ii34–ii38.

Nelson, E. C., Batalden, P. B., Huber, T. P., Mohr, J. J., Godfrey, M. M., Headrick, L. A., et al. (2002). Microsystems in health care: Part 1. Learning from high-performing front-line clinical units. *Joint Commission Journal of Quality and Safety, 28,* 472–493.

Peters, T. J., & Waterman, R. H. (1982). In search of excellence: Lessons learned from America's best run companies. New York: Harper & Row.

Schein, E. (1992). *Organizational culture and leadership.* San Francisco: Jossey-Bass.

Simons, T. (2002). Behavioral integrity: The perceived alignment between managers' words and deeds as a research focus. *Organization Science, 13*(1), 18–35.

White, R. K., & Lippit, R. (1960). *Autocracy and democracy: An experimental inquiry.* New York: Harper and Brothers.

Zand, D. E. (1972). Trust and managerial problem solving. *Administrative Science Quarterly, 17*(2), 229–239.

CHAPTER 3

Leadership IQ: An Evidence-Based Organizing Schema

Dori Taylor Sullivan and Emmett C. Murphy

CHAPTER QUESTIONS

1. What is Leadership IQ and how was it discovered?
2. How can Leadership IQ enhance the actions and outcomes of clinical leaders?
3. How can clinical leaders begin to assess their own Leadership IQ?

INTRODUCTION

Leadership IQ is the second component or lens recommended for use in our model of effective leadership. Leadership IQ (LIQ) is a description of behaviors or roles observed in highly effective leaders that were identified and studied through an extensive research study. Because it was derived from a study and provides a detailed yet practical idea of best-performing leaders' practices, LIQ was selected as one of the core model elements.

This chapter briefly describes the LIQ research process, then introduces the elements of LIQ and hallmarks of its use for leadership development, and closes with suggested application exercises to boost your LIQ.

LEADERSHIP IQ: A USEFUL FRAMEWORK

Practicing clinical leaders may be overwhelmed with the plethora of leadership theories, approaches, and assessments that pepper management publications. While most have some value, the real-world challenge is to figure out what knowledge or theory applies in each situation faced. Perhaps most important leaders must determine how their time is spent on a daily if not hourly basis to achieve the best results in a constantly changing environment. Last,

Figure 3.1   Leadership IQ At-A-Glance

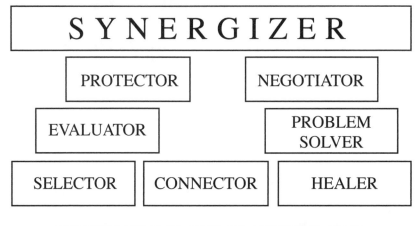

GUIDING PRINCIPLES

leaders interested in developing their skills and performance would like some assurance that the recommendations provided actually work! Leadership IQ is the second lens or theory in the model for clinical leadership presented in this book that we recommend using to better understand and respond to common leadership changes. Figure 3.1 provides an illustration of Leadership IQ.

Leadership IQ (Murphy, 1996) provides a framework of "leadership intelligence" that is derived from the practices of 1,029 highly effective leaders in a sample of more than 18,000 from all major industries. What was learned from these best practice leaders was translated into a theory of leadership behavior and a related personal development process. You can use LIQ to decide how to respond to leadership situations or challenges as well as to assess your personal skills in LIQ principles and roles. Leadership IQ boasts a cadre of worldwide supporters who embraced its practical yet incredibly rich approach to leadership. Education and development programs based on LIQ, and its subsequent iterations and applications (including team IQ, board IQ, and others), have been tested extensively with health care leaders, with high levels of participant and organizational satisfaction. We are confident that you will find LIQ of value as you continue to develop your leadership practice.

Table 3.1 is an LIQ checklist for you to complete to get a sense of your stronger and weaker skills in the LIQ guiding principles and role areas. We recommend that you look over the checklist before reading the chapter. Then return to and complete the checklist.

Table 3.1 Leadership IQ Checklist for Clinical Leaders

Use the following scoring system for each answer below. Place an X in the appropriate column. Indicate the extent to which you believe in the following statements using the scale below:

1 = Do not believe
2 = Believe somewhat
3 = Strongly believe

Section 1. LIQ Guiding Principles

	1	2	3
The quality of individuals' work and their focus on their work is what leads to achievement and recognition in most cases.			
The best solutions are often creative but direct and simple.			
It is powerful to acknowledge what you don't know with others because learning is a lifelong endeavor.			
The customer or focus of our services must always be at the center of our consideration.			
It is important to be committed to our work, our colleagues, and our beliefs.			
Choosing to see the glass as half full not half empty promotes positive outlooks.			
People are responsible for the choices they make in life along with the consequences of those choices.			

Section 2. LIQ Roles

Use the following scoring system for each answer below. Place an X in the appropriate column. Consider the extent to which you as a leader are able to perform the following activities using the scale below:

1 = Do rarely and not well at all
2 = Do moderately well and some of the time
3 = Do well and most of the time

	1	2	3
Select the right people for a job or task.			
Communicate effectively and connect with individuals and groups.			
Proactively identify and solve important problems.			

Table 3.1 Leadership IQ Checklist for Clinical Leaders (*continued*)

	1	2	3
Evaluate performance and progress of individuals and projects.			
Negotiate successful resolutions to conflicts.			
Recognize and deal with the negative feelings associated with change or other events in the workplace.			
Identify and respond to threats or crises to protect the organization/unit and its culture.			
Promote synergized efforts that result in people working together and achieving more than would have been predicted.			
Comments:			

THE LEADERSHIP IQ RESEARCH

The study of leadership that generated LIQ began in the early 1990s, directed by Dr. Emmett C. Murphy using databases that reflected the beliefs and practices of more than 18,000 leaders within 562 business, health care, and public service organizations. A technique called *known groups* that involves soliciting many opinions to identify people who most exemplify certain qualities (in this case leaders who are thought to do the job very well) was used to identify high-performing leaders. A sample of 1,029 leaders (designated as workleaders) from all levels met the criteria for inclusion that included acknowledgment by superiors, peers, and subordinates for being highly effective as well as consistent achievers of organizational goals, including financial performance for their units of responsibility.

Six major findings of the research were identified. First, leadership can be defined and measured as a form of intelligence—and workleaders are not "born" but "made" as they develop their knowledge and skills. Second, observations suggested that the separation of workers from leaders is arbitrary and that in the most effective organizations every leader works and every worker

Table 3.2 LIQ Leader Roles

1. Selector
2. Connector
3. Problem Solver
4. Evaluator
5. Negotiator
6. Healer
7. Protector
8. Synergizer

leads. Third, workleaders know how to say the right thing to the right people at the right time to get work done well. The fourth insight was that workleaders used specific tools or techniques to fulfill eight specific leadership roles (Table 3.2) that are the "heart" of LIQ; these include actions benchmark leaders take to:

- Select the right people.
- Connect them to the right cause.
- Solve problems that arise.
- Evaluate progress toward objectives.
- Negotiate resolutions to conflicts.
- Heal the wounds inflicted by change.
- Protect their cultures from the perils of crisis.
- Synergize all stakeholders in a way that enables them to achieve improvement together (Murphy, 1996, p. 4).

The fifth research finding suggests that the most effective workleaders have mastered all eight roles and thus achieve a "synergistic kick" that may be described as a gestalt; that is, the resulting performance is more than the sum of its separate parts within the roles. And sixth, it was determined that workleaders had very different patterns of time utilization—they spent most of their time in proactive problem-solving activities rather than on routine or maintenance responsibilities.

LIQ Guiding Principles

A final insight occurred after the research was substantially completed and resulted from interacting with this highly effective group of leaders. Workleaders were observed to consistently obey seven guiding principles in everything they do and say (Murphy, 1996, p. 13). These principles appear in Table 3.3.

Table 3.3   LIQ Guiding Principles

- Be an achiever
- Be pragmatic
- Practice strategic humility
- Be customer-focused
- Be committed
- Be a learned optimist
- Be responsible

Murphy noted (1996, p. 13) that individuals with high LIQ scores have "mastered the equivalent of a liberal arts education in the practical realities of human behavior and . . . have learned how to make business and society work." The LIQ guiding principles incorporate personal and professional integrity, one of the most widely cited characteristics of successful leaders (Annison & Wilford, 1998; Barker, 1990; Drucker, 1999; Freiberg & Freiberg, 1996; Senge, 1990; and Studer, 2003). However, each guiding principle introduces a unique and important dimension when considering the behavior of health care leaders.

The *achievement* paradigm promotes a focus on the work and individuals' accomplishment of that work as opposed to favoritism and personal connections, which leads to positive results and enhanced, realistic self-esteem. The *pragmatic* approach of effective workleaders is one of the most effective ways to link to coworkers at all levels because most people value a practical yet ingenious solution to a problem versus an overly complex process, or in common language driving a nail with a sledge hammer. As you learn more about complexity science and health care leadership, these themes of relative simplicity and setting direction but not specifics appear many times. Effective leaders analyze a situation and set a course of action that is clear, direct, and likely to work. *Strategic humility* similarly endears leaders to others through a willingness to acknowledge their lack of knowledge and/or a need for others' contributions while promoting individual, group, and organizational learning (Senge, 1990).

The guiding principle that reflects *customer focus* may be one of the most important in distinguishing high-performing from mediocre or low-performing leaders. Workleaders consistently and seemingly intuitively provide or solicit customer perspectives and needs, rather than considering them as an afterthought. Workleaders have a palpable connection to customers as essential partners in every endeavor. This synergy with customers promotes organizational behaviors and outcomes that fulfill and even anticipate customer needs and desires, often leading to competitive advantage. The chapter on customer needs addresses this critical principle in detail.

Workleaders are viewed as *committed* to the people around them, the organization, and themselves. As we noted before, coworkers gravitate toward transformational leaders who emit signals that energize and encourage others to renew their loyalty to the organization or unit. The impact of commitment with *learned optimism* is a double win. Effective leaders learn to be optimistic not by ignoring the negatives but by choosing to focus on the realistic, positive elements of any situation. The final guiding principle of *accepting responsibility* underlies all those previously stated. When responsibility for work, or life, is totally embraced, there is a sense of internal control and the sense that we can make it happen rather than letting things happen to us. These seven guiding principles comprise the core belief system of the workleaders studied. These core beliefs are consistently exhibited in the eight LIQ roles.

Many managers develop strength in these areas along their pathway to leadership roles and through emulating positive role models. People in leadership roles should consciously assess their values, attitudes, and behaviors related to each of the guiding principles. You have likely recognized that the guiding principles reflect the type of leader that others wish to follow. We recommend that whenever possible you highlight these principles in analyzing and responding to situations, both individually and as part of team discussions.

The Eight Workleader Roles of LIQ

The effective leaders whose behavior spawned LIQ demonstrated expertise in each of the roles, leading to the synergistic kick referenced earlier and named in the eighth role. A hallmark of these benchmark leaders was the repeated use of relatively simple tools or approaches to deal with even complex situations. It has been said that complex problems require simple solutions. The use of consistent approaches leads to predictable leadership behavior that others grow to count on and expect, thus lowering the anxiety associated with the unknown.

We briefly describe each of the eight workleader roles but we encourage readers to access the LIQ monograph (Murphy, 1996) for a full presentation of the roles and specific tools recommended for use within each role.

The book emphasizes the use of scripts for each LIQ role to increase consistency and effectiveness. The tools associated with each role provide strategies for effective leadership actions and have been tested in practice. Finally, a universal set of steps is provided as a guide to action in situations that are not easily categorized into the eight LIQ roles.

The Selector

The selector role in LIQ is considered first since it is essential to have a good fit between individual goals and abilities and the goals and needs of the organization and its customers. One of LIQ's significant contributions is to position the selection function as being always for the customer. Another contribution is giving the four aspects of selection that include initial hiring or assignment, reselection, debriefing when employees leave through voluntary turnover or nonperformance-related issues, and separation or termination.

When hiring into a position, it is crucial that leaders analyze how the position should be configured to maximize its focus on priority elements. In Chapter 12 we discuss work analysis in greater detail. Once this analysis has occurred, it is easier to specify the ideal candidate. Murphy (1996) along with others (Freiberg & Freiberg, 1996) suggested that in many cases we hire individuals for their technical skills or resume qualifications rather than their core attributes, attitudes, and values. The Southwest Airlines success story (Freiberg & Freiberg, 1996) coined the term "hire for attitude" to clearly communicate that organization's belief in the importance of values and attitudes as essential hiring criteria. It is recommended that only the absolute minimum technical specifications be listed—and then hire the best personality for the job and train for specific functions.

Too often leaders think of selection only in relation to new hires. In fact, for many leaders the other three aspects of selection are equally or more important in creating a highly functioning work group. Reselection refers to the periodic assessment of individuals in terms of their ongoing fit with assigned roles and responsibilities. Both organizations and individuals change over time in subtle and obvious ways, some of which enhance performance and fit while others lead to declining performance and/or job dissatisfaction. In LIQ, reselection does not mean dismissal or the practice of eliminating all positions and then asking people to reapply. It does mean that leaders consciously and systematically engage individuals in a process to assess their fit over time as well as changing preferences for reward and recognition activities. Often creative options can be crafted to modify a role or responsibilities or redeploy individuals to better serve customers as well as meet worker preferences.

When an employee makes the decision to leave, incredibly valuable information about the work unit, its processes, and people—including the leader—lies in the hands of those leaving. This essential information must be captured into the leader's feedback loops for proactive assessment and improvement purposes. It also provides the context for recognizing contributions and reinforcing self-esteem rather than the typical rapid exit without communication that many workers experience. Proceeding in this manner promotes the core values and LIQ guiding principles learned from benchmark leaders. Last, when a decision has been made to separate an employee, LIQ provides a scripted approach that combines strategies to maintain esteem while clearly delivering the termination message.

Once the leader has made the important selection decisions and any desired personnel changes, it is time to focus on the connector role to foster individual and team achievement.

The Connector

As complexity science also informs us of the need to build relationships among key people, the goal of the connector role within LIQ is to build and enhance relationships through highly targeted and effective communication. Accomplishing this requires the assessment of individual and/or group levels of commitment and preferred communication styles across the work team. There are many models of business and general communication available; however, LIQ again distinguishes itself by proposing specific assessment tools and solutions that leaders can use immediately after becoming aware of them.

The connector role tools highlight the need to assess individual and group communication styles and preferences as well as the level of commitment, both of which influence the leader's communication strategies. The most effective leaders have developed their assessment strategies in these areas and enhanced their communication styles so that they can tailor their messages for each audience to promote acceptance and understanding. As we are all well aware, the ability of leaders to communicate and connect to others is one of the most important leadership determinants.

While there are several options for assessing individual communication styles and preferences, one of the tools in LIQ is particularly useful due to its face value and logic. The relationship styles grid (Murphy, 1996, p. 66) defines four types of relators: rational, functional, intuitive, and personal. Rational relators are characterized as analytical, factual, and technical. Functional relators are described as planners, organizers, and controlled. Intuitive relators are defined as conceptual, visionary, and creative. And finally, personal relators are seen as sensitive, subjective, and verbal.

The contribution of the LIQ relationship styles grid is a simple yet compelling organizing framework that allows leaders to determine style preferences and respond to them with a few simple observations or questions. The types of role tools contained in LIQ are sensitive to the real-time constraints faced by managers, and recommended strategies are time efficient as well as results focused. The connector role reminds managers of the critical importance of tailoring communications to each audience so they not only hear but embrace the message.

The Problem Solver

The simply stated goal of the problem solver role is to produce desired results. The LIQ research clearly showed that benchmark leaders spent more time in problem-solving activities than did less effective leaders (more on this later in the section on time distribution among the roles). Further, it was evident that the most successful leaders engaged in proactive problem solving, scanning the environment, and "connecting" with staff to detect issues and take action early.

A set of recommended steps along with tools is designed to elicit relevant data and analyze that data with critical new eyes (problem transformation) then engage workers in the problem-solving process (problem analysis and solutions worksheet).

During problem-solving activities, the leader has the opportunity to promote focus on the major customer(s) while positively influencing the resolution of issues and achieving improvements designed by the individual or work group members. Instead of problems being deposited on the manager's desk, early indicators of problems (and many times opportunities) are addressed and resolved. As with other roles, the use of a script or step-by-step approach promotes consistent and productive leader behavior.

The Evaluator

Although evaluation is a critical part of every manager's responsibilities, it is easy to back away from because many people feel uncomfortable judging the work of others, especially recognizing their own imperfections and weaknesses. The goal of the LIQ evaluator role is to enhance individual performance. The evaluator role in LIQ emphasizes customer focus and personal responsibility in promoting high-quality care and services.

Benchmark workleaders were more willing to recognize high performance and had wider variations of ratings among staff, reflecting their commitment to honest communication to foster improvement. These high but not unrealistic expectations foster a positive work environment that in turn attracts other high performers.

Using contemporary human resource performance evaluation tools and techniques, highly effective leaders assure that evaluation tools are customer-focused, relevant, balanced, and reliable. This, and other related human resource topics, are discussed in Chapters 12 and 13.

The Negotiator

The role of the negotiator in the LIQ framework is to develop consensus to better serve customers, a notion that flies in the face of some popular approaches to negotiation that propose winning as the ultimate goal. The concept of consensus is also critical to this definition, as it promotes positive commit-ment to a course of action among potentially diverse constituencies while building trust, relationships, and self-esteem. Consensus may be defined as "the process of achieving synergy by combining the strengths and visions of each party in a new way to achieve something neither could have achieved alone." This type of consensus may also be described as collaboration. In con-trast, compromise means that both or all parties give up some thing(s) of sig-nificance in relatively equal proportions to achieve a solution. Most people do not find compromise a very fulfilling outcome and even its definition does lit-tle to promote excitement or satisfaction. Consensus speaks to possibilities and new creations, thus it is energizing and positive. A detailed discussion of conflict management is contained in Chapter 13.

The general steps for successful negotiating include establishing purpose, identifying customer needs, developing a solution, testing the solution, identify-ing barriers, overcoming barriers, and taking action together. Thus, negotiation becomes something done for the customer, refocusing away from individual or work group preferences and minimizing the impact of self-interests in decision making. For most leaders, negotiation is a daily event and a way of life rather than an episodic event so solid ability in this area is essential for success.

The Healer

The next two LIQ roles tend to initially puzzle first-time readers, yet upon examination their integral contributions are easily seen. The healer role seeks to address the impact of individual, group, or organizational "health" prob-lems, recognizing that the leader must be able to diagnose and prescribe ac-tions to address these potentially disruptive situations. Healing may be re-quired on an individual basis for a worker experiencing life stresses as well as for surfacing and designing healing strategies for a work group that has expe-rienced a significant change such as reorganization.

The LIQ approach highlights the need for leaders to be familiar with behav-ioral, attitudinal, and physical indicators of distress or dysfunction, along with a list of common diagnoses that may call for a healing intervention. As with other workleader roles, a proactive approach is recommended.

A hallmark of the healer role is the positive context for recognizing and in-tervening in situations, which in other writings on management might be in-cluded in a section on performance problems or morale issues. The health care environment has experienced dramatic and destructive changes under the guise of improvement that have had a significant impact on individuals and de-partments or groups. The healer role promotes enhanced sensitivity to events that affect workers in ways that call for healing.

Benchmark leaders differed significantly from their lower performing peers in early recognition and interventions to promote healing in the workplace. The healer role not only promotes solutions for the individual or group to enhance performance and positive feelings but also demonstrates consistency with the guiding principles and builds commitment through caring for others.

The Protector

While many leaders are very committed to their organizations, it is doubtful they would describe themselves as organizational protectors! Yet that is the essence of this LIQ role. The protector diagnoses and responds to threats to organizational well-being through the tools of risk assessment and conflict management.

Risk assessment gathers the necessary information to gauge the depth and type of risk the unit or organization may or does face. Leaders are charged with anticipating the risk and identifying its type, planning to take charge, and learning from the risk. Since serious risks may be viewed as a crisis, and crisis tends to create interpersonal conflicts, conflict management skills are highly important. Leaders are strongly advised to personally assess the risk in crisis situations, in contrast to other approaches. Many a manager has failed to act in a crisis situation because he was assured by others that the risk was not severe or was resolved. Another key element of the LIQ protector role speaks to measuring solutions against the values and mission of the organization, often easily defined by what is in best service to the customer.

As with the negotiator role, the focus is always on serving the customer, not personal or professional gains or losses. Unmanaged conflicts against a backdrop of organizational threat is a formula for real disaster, thus highly effective leaders work hard to hone and maintain their skills as organizational protectors.

The Synergizer

"Through the role of synergizer, workleaders impress the principles of self-determination and its corollary, personal responsibility, deeply into the consciousness of their organizations. This reflects the seminal characteristic of the 1,029 exceptional leaders identified by both colleagues and customers in [our] study population of more than 18,000 people." (Murphy, 1996, p. 223)

The synergizer's function is to create a whole greater than the sum of its parts through a seemingly effortless deployment of the right words to the right people at the right time to serve the customer. In describing the synergizer's role, LIQ notes that choosing change approaches that reflect the transformational leadership values of vision, collaboration, commitment, and self-determination helps effective leaders actively adapt to and invent change.

Since change is a constant in organizations, leaders must constantly assess the need for change and promote systematic self-improvement among all to prepare for the challenges of tomorrow.

In discussing the synergizer role, a generic formula called the seven-step guide (Murphy, 1996, p. 230) may be adapted for general use. Although many leadership challenges will be situations that fit into the other LIQ roles, leaders must be prepared for any scenario. These seven steps used by benchmark leaders that provide an overall approach to improvement include:

- Establishing context (What is the challenge and vision for meeting it?).
- Measuring mission effectiveness.
- Identifying opportunities for improvement.
- Mobilizing support.
- Taking action.
- Measuring results.
- Improving continuously.

According to Dr. Murphy (1996, p. 245), the LIQ roles and especially the synergizer

> address the visionary, strategic, and tactical objectives of leadership in a way that integrates large-scale change with everyday life. For a workleader, change is a seamless spiral from selection, connection, problem solving, evaluation, negotiation, healing, and protection to the culminating act of synergizing. This continuity of practice lies at the heart of the workleader's integrity and power to attain incomparable levels of achievement.

Time Allocation Among the Workleader Roles

The LIQ research assessed how benchmark leaders spend their time across the eight leadership roles. The most effective workleaders spent most of their time in the problem solver role, anticipating and actively seeking issues to be resolved before they became crises. The next most significant block of time was devoted to the other workleader roles, with maintenance or routine administrative functions allocated the least amount of time. Highly effective leaders retain their focus and spend their most precious resource—time—in the areas that will mobilize the team to achieve organizational goals. It is sad but true that many managers do not have an accurate picture of how they spend their time, and may be driven away from priority actions by bureaucratic demands. Benchmark leaders exhibit strategies to accomplish the necessary administrative tasks without allowing them to compromise the key leadership roles and functions. We look at managing personal resources including time in Chapter 6.

Assessing Organizational Work Practices as a Context for LIQ

When using LIQ for individual or group performance development or for assessing a given situation, the climate or culture of the specific organization must be taken into account because the culture is the context within which we as leaders practice our craft. The LIQ assessment notes the influence of organizational culture factors such as core values, commitment to customers, work focus and efficiency, quality of service, quality of life, and readiness for change, among others. This organizational context is then used to interpret and plan individual leadership actions or development with the goal of enhancing or changing organizational culture to support best leadership practices.

Finally, the influence of the overall health care environment must be taken into account as changing issues and practices often create significant organizational culture impacts or adjustments to positively adapt and continue organizational success.

BOOSTING YOUR LIQ

Leadership IQ (Murphy, 1996) provides a tested and straightforward conceptualization of what leaders need to do and how to do it. In addition to the tools included, there is a self-assessment available with answers and detailed interpretation guidelines.

It is critically important that clinical leaders think through what their roles are, consciously allocate their time and resources to the most important ones, and develop efficient and effective "scripts" or methods of dealing with commonly occurring events. This not only enhances performance but can increase confidence and decrease stress. Consideration of the specific context of the organization's culture and values provides the context for using LIQ in different institutions.

The LIQ framework is used throughout the remainder of this book to illustrate how the systematic use of the LIQ lens or theory can help clinical managers achieve their best outcomes.

APPLICATION EXERCISES

1. Refer back to Table 3.1 and answer the questions provided to do a quick check of your current inclinations related to LIQ Guiding Principles and Roles. Discuss your answers with a mentor.

2. Think of a recent situation that you as a clinical leader had to deal with that relates to each of the eight workleader roles. Would using the LIQ roles to anticipate and respond improve your actions in these situations?

REFERENCES

Anniston, M. H., & Wilford, D. S. (1998). *Trust matters: New directions in health care leadership.* San Francisco: Jossey-Bass.

Barker, Anne. A. M. (1992). *Transformational leadership in nursing: A vision for the future.* Baltimore, MD: Williams & Wilkins.

Drucker, P. F. (1999). *Management challenges for the 21st century.* New York: Harper-Collins.

Freiberg, K., & Freiberg, J. (1996). *Nuts!: Southwest Airlines' crazy recipe for business and personal success.* Austin, TX: Bard.

Murphy, E. C. (1996). *Leadership IQ: A personal development process based on a scientific study of a new generation of leaders.* New York: John Wiley & Sons.

Senge, P. (1990). *The fifth discipline: The art and practice of the learning organization.* New York: Currency Doubleday.

Studer, Q. (2003). *Hardwiring excellence.* Gulf Breeze, FL: Fire Starter.

CHAPTER 4

Leadership Development Through Mentorship and Professional Development Planning

Anne M. Barker

────── **CHAPTER QUESTIONS** ──────

1. Why is it important for me to have a mentor?
2. How do I select a mentor?
3. What should I expect of the relationship as it evolves?
4. What is networking and why should I do it?
5. How do I identify my professional development needs and make a plan to achieve them?

INTRODUCTION

The mentor-mentee relationship is a very special one between two individuals. The benefits of having a mentor, or more than one, are well documented and you should consider them as you decide to find a mentor or enhance the role a mentor plays in your career. This chapter can help you evaluate the mentoring relationship and provide a structure for working with your mentor.

Research regarding mentorship shows that individuals who have a mentor, as compared to those not having a mentor, have:

- Increased job satisfaction.
- Higher salaries.
- Enhanced self-esteem and confidence.
- Greater opportunities for promotion and advancement.
- Enhanced role socialization.
- A definitive career plan (Grindell, 2003).

MENTORSHIP MODEL

From the many definitions of a mentor, for this book we have adopted the classic definition proposed by Vance (1982). She defines a mentor as an experienced person who guides and nurtures a less experienced person (the mentee). The mentor is someone who inspires, instructs, nurtures, and encourages the mentee. Vance states that the mentoring relationship is a helping relationship that is special, emotional, intense, and enduring as opposed to shorter term and less intense relationships such as preceptor, sponsor, role model, or peer.

Figure 4.1 illustrates our model of mentorship, which we have devised through a review of the literature and our own personal experiences of having a mentor and being a mentor. The relationship between the mentor and mentee can best be described as a partnership. In this partnership there is a congruency between the expertise and organizational connections of the mentor and the learning needs of the mentee. Further, since the goal of being mentored is to increase your transformational leadership skills, the mentor must be a transformational leader role model. As a result of the relationship and interactions between the two, the mentee is energized for self-reflection, learning, and action, leading to professional role development and growth.

At the heart of this relationship, there must be mutual trust and respect and open communications (Klein & Dickenson-Hazzard, 2000). The mentee will be disclosing sensitive information, exposing weaknesses, and discussing lack of skills and competence in job-related areas. Thus, the mentee must feel that he or she can be open and honest and, in return, expect confidential, nonjudgmental, and sensitive feedback from the mentor.

STAGES OF THE MENTOR-MENTEE RELATIONSHIP

The mentor-mentee relationship ideally exists over a long period of time and therefore goes through several stages (Anderson et al. 2002). Each stage is discussed below. You can use this information to understand what to expect from a mentor-mentee relationship, or if you already have a mentor, use the information to assess your relationship.

Stage One: Selecting a Mentor and Determining Expectations

Mentee-mentor relationships are formed in health care organizations in one of two ways, formally or informally. Some organizations have formal, structured mentorship programs established to assist new managers in learning their role. If such a program exists in your organization, you should take full advantage of it. The benefit of a formal mentorship program is that it provides

Figure 4.1   The Barker-Sullivan Model of Mentor Partnerships

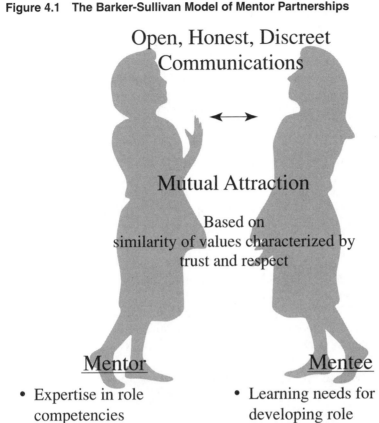

Open, Honest, Discreet
Communications

Mutual Attraction

Based on
similarity of values characterized by
trust and respect

<u>Mentor</u>

- Expertise in role competencies
- Transformational leader
- Skills as a mentor

<u>Mentee</u>

- Learning needs for developing role competencies and leadership skills

energized

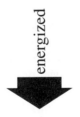

- Self reflection
- Learning
- Action

structure and well-defined expectations for both parties, as well as deploys organizational resources, particularly time, for the ongoing development of the relationship (Anderson et al., 2002).

Having a formal mentorship program does not preclude your having other informal mentor relationship(s) initiated by you. In fact, we believe that informal mentor relationships are best because at the heart of the mentor-mentee relationship is an attraction of both people whose personality and values fit. Informal mentor-mentee relationships happen because both the mentor and mentee wish to work together and share mutual respect and admiration. This may or may not happen when one is assigned a mentor in a formal program.

Either mentor or mentee can initiate the relationship. For the purposes of this book, however, we are suggesting that you seek out the appropriate person(s) to mentor you.

There are many considerations as you decide who to ask to mentor you. We offer several guidelines to assist you in identifying appropriate individuals. First, you may find that there are several people who you would consider as mentors. Each of these individuals can bring something different to your professional growth and development; therefore, do not rule out having more than one mentor.

Second, we do not recommend that you choose your direct supervisor or a potential supervisor. There are several reasons for this, the most important being that since your supervisor serves as your evaluator you may be reluctant to be vulnerable and share what you see as your weaknesses in fear that they will turn up on an official evaluation. However, to be an effective clinical leader, you do need to establish an effective and appropriate relationship with your supervisor. Having a mentor can help you with this relationship and contribute to your professional growth and learning.

A third consideration is whether to ask someone within or outside your own organization to serve as your mentor. The pros of having an internal mentor are that the person knows the organization, can help you make connections, can observe your behaviors and outcomes, and may get indirect feedback about your performance from others. On the other hand, a mentor external to your organization can offer new insights and different ways of doing things and can help you make connections outside the organization.

A final consideration is whether to use a peer mentor or someone in a position advanced from yours, other than your supervisor. The advantages of having a mentor from your peers are that they are experiencing the issues and needs of the role in a way similar to you. Their network of connections may be more appropriate to you. A mentor at a higher level in the organization, however, can provide a broader view of the organization and a different level of connections with others.

In summary, we encourage you to consider having more than one mentor representing other disciplines, both genders, cultural and generational diversity, and professionals who work in other organizations. Table 4.1 is a checklist for you to use in selecting someone to mentor you. The first six questions focus on the person's leadership skills and role expertise. If you answer "no" to any of these questions, then we recommend reconsidering the person as your mentor. However, you may find that they have several important skills

Table 4.1   Mentor Selection Checklist

Name of Potential Mentor: Brief explanation of why you are considering this person:			
Desired Characteristic	**Yes**	**No**	**Don't Know**
1. Does the person have the expert knowledge and skills in the competencies that you need to develop?			
2. Is the person a transformational leader by action and by example?			
3. Does this person have the ability to guide, coach, and teach you?			
4. Is the person respected in the organization?			
5. Does the person have access to important organizational information and can he or she help you to direct attention on important issues?			
6. Does the person have a network of influential people and is willing to assist you to be visible, credible, and accepted by others in the organization?			
7. Is the person willing to work collaboratively with you?			
8. Is the person willing to spend the time and energy required for the development of this relationship?			
9. Are you comfortable with this person and trust him or her to hold confidentiality?			
10. Is the person able to provide you with negative as well as positive feedback?			
11. Can the person help you identify what you need to learn and provide the structure for learning activities?			
Summary Statement:			

you wish to learn and that in doing the assessment you become aware of what they can and cannot offer you. The last five questions relate to the person's ability to be an effective mentor.

After selecting a mentor(s) the next step is to establish ground rules. Borges and Smith (2004) provide a set of strategies to set up expectations for the relationship in this very early stage. First, they suggest setting up the details of when, where, and how long meetings will take place and what other forms of communication, such as e-mail, you will use. Second, the mentee should write down long-term career goals/vision and use this as a starting point for discussion and planning. The last strategy is to develop specific professional learning goals and personal goals. In the next section of this chapter we provide you with tools for assessing your developmental needs and a form for documenting your plans for meeting these needs and progress toward your goals. In this process the mentee should also consider life goals such as salary, health, family, spiritual needs, and so forth. We believe that a clinical manager must lead a balanced and happy life to be an effective transformational leader. A mentor can help you set and pay attention to your personal goals and help you balance them with your professional goals.

Stage Two: Development of Role Competencies

In stage two the mentee works on developmental goals by engaging in specific learning activities, with the guidance and support of the mentor. The mentor serves as teacher, advisor, facilitator, coach, and sounding board (Anderson et al., 2002). During this time the mentor connects the mentee to appropriate people both inside and outside the organization and helps the mentee understand the organizational culture and political realities of getting the job done.

Stage Three: Growing Independence

As time progresses the mentee grows in confidence, gains the necessary knowledge and skills to be an effective transformational leader, and demonstrates the attainment of the role competencies. At this point the mentee begins to seek independence, and the mentor role changes to consultant, giving advice only when asked (Anderson et al., 2002).

Stage Four: The Dissolution of the Relationship

In the last stage the mentee is ready to move on from the relationship and no longer needs the mentor's advice and support. However, often an enduring friendship and colleagueship evolves and is maintained over the course of many years (Anderson et al., 2002).

MENTORSHIP VERSUS NETWORKING

Networking is interacting with individuals within and outside the organization to share ideas, information, and experiences, and to give and get advice. In contrast to mentoring, networking has less sustained interactions with others and is less structured. Having a network of people is as important for your professional development as it is to have a mentor.

For networking to be effective, you need to reflect on your networking needs and set up processes to ensure that you interact with people who can contribute to your professional growth and development. First of all, think about people in your organization who you believe can provide you with good insights about the organization, whose personality and values fit yours, whose communication style is compatible with yours, and who might be willing to share with you. In turn, think about people in your organization with whom you could share your experiences and ideas. You should think about this broadly and include other disciplines and peers. Next, you simply need to make contact with these people by asking them for coffee, to have lunch with you, or to stay after a meeting for a few minutes just to talk or to ask for their advice about a specific issue. As you establish a relationship with others, phone calls and e-mail will assist you in maintaining contact even when you are busy. The key here is to be attentive about developing the networks, rather than just letting the relationships emerge. Further, you and the person you network with should establish guidelines for confidentiality, being clear what information can and cannot be shared.

Besides having a network within your organization, you should also establish a network of contacts outside the organization. Most often this occurs through your professional organizations and meetings. Just as you think through whom your internal network should be the same should happen for establishing a network of people who are not in your organization. Make contact with others and establish a structure for maintaining the contact over time.

A MODEL OF CAREER DEVELOPMENT

In the next section of this chapter, you will engage in a process for assessing your career development needs and planning for continual growth. These activities should provide a structure for you and your mentor to begin your initial work together. Our goal in having you engage in this activity is for you to develop certain capabilities, including:

- Engaging in self-reflection and self-awareness.
- Enhancing your self-confidence.

- Learning to take a broad systematic view of health care and your organization.
- Learning to work effectively within your organization and with others.
- Developing the ability to think critically and creatively.
- Engaging in experimental learning.

Klein (2004) presents a model of career development that provides a useful framework for reflecting on all your career development needs. Most leadership development programs place an emphasis on the development of individual skills and competencies and learning how the organization works while ignoring the vision and values of the individual and the organization. This model presents a more holistic view; the tools presented here were developed using this framework.

Table 4.2 has four quadrants to consider in looking at career development. Individual and collective aspects are placed along the vertical axis while internal and external aspects are placed along the horizontal axis. Individual aspects are things you need to consider about yourself whereas collective aspects deal with the organization and the larger world.

Quadrants 1 and 2 list individual aspects of your career, internal and external, respectively. Quadrant 1 is the internal or self-aspects. In this area you reflect on your individual values, purposes, and the personal meaning that leadership and

Table 4.2   Model of Career Development

	Internal	**External**
Individual	**Quadrant 1** **Self** • Values • Purposes • Personal meaning	**Quadrant 2** **Your Behaviors** • Competencies • Skills • Knowledge • Leadership traits
Collective	**Quadrant 3** **Organizational Culture** • Vision • Shared values • Shared purpose • Relationships	**Quadrant 4** **The Environment** • Organizational structures and systems • Technology • The health care delivery system

Source: Klein, E. (2002, First Quarter). Missing something in your career? *Reflections on Nursing Leadership*, 41–42.

your profession have for you. In quadrant 2 the external individual aspects of career development (behaviors) reside and include the competencies and skills needed to perform your job or to obtain advanced positions.

Quadrants 3 and 4 attend to the collective aspects of your career, both internal and external. In quadrant 3, the internal collective aspects of organizational culture include consideration of the shared values, shared purposes, and relationships that affect how you relate to others in the organization. Quadrant 4, the environment, includes the organizational structures and systems, policies and procedures, and technology in the organization.

It is useful to study Table 4.2 to gain a full understanding of your career development needs. No one quadrant stands on its own. For instance, if you look at both individual and collective internal factors, you realize that your values and beliefs as an individual must be consistent with the values and purposes of the organization. Likewise, if you look at the external factor, the competencies and skills you develop must be pertinent to and useful for the environment in which you work. These activities can maximize the chances of a good fit between you and the organization, increasing your satisfaction with your role.

PROCESS FOR CAREER DEVELOPMENT PLANNING

Using the career development model, we suggest that you engage in a four-step career development planning process (Donner & Wheeler, 2001). Tables 4.3 and 4.4 give two tools to help you integrate these steps with the model:

- Scan the environment (Table 4.3)
- Complete a self-assessment (Table 4.3)
- Create a career vision (Table 4.3)
- Develop a career plan (Table 4.4)

The first section of Table 4.3 asks you to scan the environment and look at the organizational culture and the environmental considerations (quadrants 3 and 4) discussed in the model. As you do this, you will be able to understand your developmental needs in a broad context of the overall environment of health care and your organization.

The second section of Table 4.3 is a self-assessment (quadrants 1 and 2) where you are asked to assess your values and beliefs, your leadership skills, and your skills and knowledge related to each of the seven role competencies. These are:

- Identifying and meeting customer needs and expectations.
- Participating in the development and implementation of the strategic plan and organizational vision.

Table 4.3   Self-Assessment of Leadership Development Needs

Section 1: Scan the environment

1. What are the current realities about health care in your organization, your state, and in the nation and what are the future trends?
2. How do you see your strengths and weaknesses related to the needs of the health care environment and the organization?
3. What are the organization's vision and shared values, and how do you contribute to moving them forward? How do people in your organization relate to one another?

Section 2: Self-Assessment

1. What are your personal values about your profession, health care? How do you find meaning and purpose in your career and in your personal life?
2. What strengths/experiences/knowledge do you have to build on? Assess this for each of the eight competencies.
3. What new experiences or knowledge do you need for the future? Assess this for each of the eight competencies.
4. What are your limitations? Assess this for each of the seven competencies.
5. Based on your assessments of your leadership skills in Chapter 2, what are your developmental needs to become an effective transformational leader?

Section 3: Career Vision

1. Where do you see yourself going?
2. What is stopping you? What are you doing about it?

- Developing and managing clinical care delivery systems.
- Promoting quality improvement and building a culture of quality by managing information to monitor and measure the quality, safety, and appropriateness of care and services.
- Leading others in the workforce to provide clinically competent care.
- Marketing clinical services.
- Managing financial resources effectively and efficiently.

In the third section of Table 4.3 you are asked to write down your overall career goal and vision. This will serve as a starting point in initiating conversations with your mentor about your goals and your learning needs.

Professional Development Plan

Based on your self-assessment, Table 4.4 can be used to develop an individualized plan for competency development, leadership skill development, and

Table 4.4 Professional Development Plan

Competency	Goals	Plans	Timelines	Resources
Customer needs and expectations				
Visioning and strategic planning				
Managing care delivery				
Improving quality				
Managing information				
Leading others				
Marketing				
Managing financial outcomes				
Leadership skill development				
Network development				
Other				

55

other areas. Space is provided for goals, plans, timelines, and the resources you will use for each of the eight role competencies.

We know it is easy to pass over these activities and exercises, feeling as if you know this in your head, but we cannot stress enough that one of the keys to success is having written goals and plans and reviewing and revising them periodically. Completing these activities and exercises will help you to select a mentor who can assist with your leaning needs. Further, this self-assessment and plan should be reviewed and revised with your mentor at planned intervals and/or when you have completed a significant accomplishment.

The benefits of goal setting are:

- You will feel that your future is positive and that you have control over where you are headed.
- You know what you want and how to get there.
- You have clear targets to focus on and to guide each day's actions and commitments.
- Your daily actions will build into personal successes over time.

APPLICATION EXERCISES

1. Identify one or more individuals in your organization or outside your organization and use Table 4.1 to assess if you should approach this person about mentoring you.
2. Complete Tables 4.3 and 4.4.

REFERENCES

Anderson, M., Kroll, B., Luoma, J., Nelson, J., Sheman, K., & Surdo, J. (2002). Mentoring relationships. *Minnesota Nursing Accent, 74 (4)*.

Borges, J. R., & Smith, B. C. (June 2004). Strategies for mentoring a diverse nursing workforce. *Nurse Leader,* 45–48.

Donner, G. J., & Wheeler, M. M. (2001). Career planning and development for nurses: The time has come. *International Nursing Review, 48* (2), 79–86.

Grindell, C. G. (2003). Mentor managers. *Nephrology Nursing Journal, 30* (5), 517–522.

Klein, E. (2004). Missing something in your career? *Reflections on Nursing Leadership, 30* (1), 41–42.

Vance, C. (1982). The mentor connection. *Journal of Nursing Administration, 12* (4), 7–13.

CHAPTER 5

Complexity Science and Change: A Path to the Future

Anne M. Barker

─────── CHAPTER QUESTIONS ───────

1. What is complexity science, and how can I use it to better understand my organization?
2. What leadership strategies should I use in viewing the organization as a complex system?
3. Using the framework of complexity, what strategies can I use to foster change?

INTRODUCTION

In this chapter we discuss two similar but distinct concepts, complexity science and change. Complexity science is an increasingly popular approach for understanding the world and organizations and has the potential to revolutionize the way we understand and analyze leadership practices. This science challenges and contradicts the view we currently hold of organizations that have guided organizational thought, structures, and systems for more than a century.

Second, we look at change theory from the perspective of how we have understood and managed changes in organizations for the past decades and integrate this with complexity science. A change model that can assist you to better manage change on your clinical unit is presented.

COMPLEXITY SCIENCE: A BRIEF INTRODUCTION

Complexity science is a broad term that can be thought of as a combination of new theories and concepts about how the world works, including chaos, complexity, and quantum theories. This new way of viewing the world and organizations is in its infancy and is thought to be the new science for the 21st century. The natural sciences such as physics, biology, and mathematics (from which complexity science has arisen) have embraced this new science as the underlying assumption for how the world works. And now there is an emerging school of managerial thought that suggests that leaders need to abandon the old ways of thinking about organizations and embrace new ones using complexity science as a framework.

In this chapter we provide a synthesis and summary of the theories that are co-concepts of complexity science. We have not provided details about each of the theories and research from which complexity science has been developed. We encourage you to use the reference list at the end of the chapter for a more thorough review of the scientific underpinnings of complexity science if you have an interest. For our purposes, the discussions about and examples of complexity science relate to health care organizations, but you should appreciate that the concepts have been developed by the physical scientist and apply to a broad view of the world.

The underlying principle of complexity science is that the world is unpredictable and is fundamentally unknowable, but in the apparent disorder order and patterns can be seen. Complexity science "holds that hidden within seemingly disorganization is a deeper structure of order. What may seem random is actually part of a larger pattern" (Lanza, 2000, p. 57).

Major Concepts of Complexity Science

Much of the work in the area of complexity science has used new, abstract terminology. In this chapter we try to simplify the concepts of complexity science and avoid the jargon when possible; however, as a clinical leader, familiarity with this new language is important for communicating with and understanding others and for further readings about this topic. We have used the language when it is appropriate and have italicized important terms. In this section we present some of the major concepts of complexity science, followed by a comparison of the new business paradigm with the old paradigm, and then conclude the discussion of complexity science with a set of leadership strategies for you to use in your practice.

In summary, from the perspective of complexity science, the world is composed of many *complex adaptive systems*. These are *nonlinear* systems in which diverse agents interact with each other and are capable of undergoing spontaneous *self-organization* (Anderson, Issel, & McDaniel, 2003). Within these complex adaptive systems, *relationships and connectedness* between the agents in the systems are the most important components of the system, not the individual agents. Complex adaptive systems are *embedded* in one another and are ever-changing and adaptable, and so the world is fundamentally *unpredictable* and *uncontrollable.* Yet from this apparent *disorder, order and patterns* emerge that are governed by *simple rules.*

In the next sections we discuss each of the terms as individual concepts, but you can see from both the definition above and within each of the descriptions below these concepts are integrated and interrelated.

Complex Adaptive Systems

At the heart of complexity science are *complex adaptive systems.* The best way to understand this term is to look at the meaning of each of the three words. "Complex" denotes wide diversity and an enormous number of agents that are multidimensional and are interconnected and interactive. "Adaptive" suggests the capacity of the agents to process information and to alter or change, in other words, the ability to learn from experiences. The term "system" denotes a set of connected interdependent elements (Zimmerman, Lindberg, & Plsek, n.d.). Examples of complex adaptive systems are molecules, living things, the ecosystem, the immune system, and organizations. Further, complex adaptive systems act locally, meaning they are not controlled by a higher level of authority.

Chapter 1 introduced the concept of the clinical unit as a microsystem, which is a complex adaptive system. First of all, it is diverse, composed of a large number of diverse individuals representing different professions, gender, ages, races, and so forth. These individuals interact with each other and are dependent on one another to complete the work of the unit. The people on the clinical unit respond to the changing internal and external environment by learning together and adapting. The clinical unit acts locally with a subpopulation of clients and families or services. The daily work is not directly controlled by the CEO or others in positions of higher authority, but by the team who gives the care. As discussed in Chapter 17, senior management influences what happens at the clinical unit level but does not control it.

To add even more complexity to the clinical unit, when thinking about complex adaptive systems in health care organizations, they are not only the individuals (patients, families, providers, payers, and so forth), but also processes such as the management information system and the departments such as human resources and finance (Plsek, 2003).

Embedded Systems

Important to our understanding of complex adaptive systems is that they are *embedded* in each other (Plsek, 2003). Looking at your unit, you can view each individual staff member as a complex adaptive system embedded in a clinical unit that is also a complex adaptive system. The unit is embedded in the organization, and the organization is embedded in the health care delivery system, which, in turn, is embedded in society.

Furthermore, an individual is an agent in more than one complex adaptive system. For instance, a staff physical therapist is an agent of the unit to which she is assigned, of the physical therapy department, of a family, and so forth. This further compounds the complexity of organizations and the relationships of the individual agents in it. Further, each individual in the organization sees the organization from a unique perspective, and no one person sees the whole picture.

Self-Organization

Another important principle of complexity science is that complex adaptive systems have the ability to *self-organize*. "Self-organizing is the process by which people mutually adjust their behaviors in ways needed to cope with changing internal and external demands" (Anderson, Issel, & McDaniel, 2003, p. 13). This means that groups of individuals will form informal alliances within the organization in order to learn, grow, and adapt to the environment.

Wheatley (1994, p. 135) proposes that the self-organizing system adapts and grows guided by one rule: "It must remain consistent with itself and its past." This allows for the paradox that the organization can be creative yet still have boundaries, that change can evolve yet there will be coherence, and that both determinism (meaning that every event is determined by previous events and conditions together with the laws of nature) and free will (meaning that the individual has the freedom to originate the event) can coexist.

Relationships and Connectedness

Mutual relationships and the *connections* between the agents in complex adaptive systems are the most important elements for successful functioning of the system. This means that an organization ought not focus on individuals but on the team effort. The observable outcomes of the system are more than a sum of its parts. It is the "generative" relationships in the organization in which the interactions among parts of a complex system produce valuable, new, and unpredictable capabilities that are not inherent in any of the parts acting alone (Plsek, 2003). For instance, a successful rehabilitation unit with good patient outcomes is not the result of any one individual but of the entire multidisciplinary team of practitioners working together. This suggests that while not abandoning efforts to retain, motivate, and reward each staff member, more efforts and systems should be employed to motivate and reward the team.

Nonlinearity

The traditional worldview is one of cause and effect and that things are related to each other in a linear way. For any change in one element there is an equal change in the next. Thus, in our organizations we have attempted to control things as if they were in a straight line.

We now understand that the world is more complex and made up of primarily *nonlinear* relationships. In fact, if you look out the window, the only things you will see that are linear are man-made. Mostly, nature consists of nonlinear structures from simple curves to complex ones such as an ecosystem or the double helix DNA. What this means for organization is that a small change in one element can produce a dramatic change in another; or the opposite often occurs when a large change effort results in very little change in behaviors or outcomes (Lanza, 2000).

Unpredictability

Based on the above concepts, the result is that the world (and the organization) is *unpredictable* and consequently uncontrollable. One basic conclusion of complexity science is that "the future behavior of a system is not predictable, regardless of how accurately one knows its present state" (McDaniel, 1997, p. 24).

Further, because complex adaptive systems are extremely sensitive to their environment, the final results are unpredictable (Lanza, 2000). In practical terms, this means that you cannot take a formula or program from one organization and simply apply it to another and expect the same results.

Order and Disorder/Simple Rules

Complexity science tells us that there is order in the disorder that we observe and that there is randomness and unpredictability because of the interactions among so many complex adaptive systems, yet at the same time there are boundaries. Wheatley (1994, p. 123) describes this concept as "order without predictability." She further describes this phenomenon as the system having "infinite possibilities, wandering wherever it pleases, sampling new configurations of itself. But its wandering and experimentation respect a boundary."

In the organization this boundary is the guiding vision, strong values, and organizational beliefs. These guide the individuals to act freely based on simply expressed expectations of acceptable behavior (Wheatley, 1994, p. 133).

Traditional Business Paradigm Versus the New Business Paradigm

Our own personal experience with learning complexity science and reported experiences of students finds that this new way of looking at the world resonates with clinical leaders. Yet putting it into practice is difficult and challenging because health care organizations are primarily characterized by a traditional view of how organizations work, and people in organizations are unwilling to take risks for fear of failure as they believe they will be punished or looked upon unfavorably.

Table 5.1 compares the traditional view of organizations with the more contemporary view that is based on complexity science. The basic assumption of how organizations worked in the traditional view is that they are machinelike and mechanistic and can be controlled and are predictable. This view came from Newtonian science in which the world was viewed as material parts with forces between them governed by laws of motion. Thus, there was a firm belief in cause and effect. From this belief, organizations developed rigid organizational policies, procedures, job descriptions, and organizational charts, attempting to control organization action. In complexity science jargon, this view of managing is often referred to as *clockware*.

As we have seen, complexity science challenges this view and suggests different leadership strategies. Rather than seeing the organization as a well-oiled machine, the organization is seen as many complex adaptive systems that can adapt in unpredictable ways and have unknown potential and capabilities. Control occurs by providing meaning and connections rather than imposing rigid operational processes. This is often called *swarmware* in complexity science terminology.

The reality is that the traditional paradigm still predominates in most, if not all, health care organizations. We believe that as time progresses the concepts of complexity science will emerge and that two views will operate simultaneously until the new paradigm eventually prevails. In the meantime, these conflicting views will cause much anxiety. We suggest that you look at the organization and your unit from both perspectives using "both/and" versus "either/or thinking." This will give you better insight and lead you to better leadership strategies. An example of this is to embrace a simple rule such as, "Always being in control is not good, but being out of control is not good either."

Leadership Strategies

From our discussion of complexity science and a comparison of the new business paradigm versus the old, six major leadership strategies have been derived from the review of the literature. These strategies should be used in concert with and as a complement to other strategies discussed in this book:

- Strategy 1: Fostering Relationships
- Strategy 2: Viewing the Organization Through the Lens of Complexity
- Strategy 3: Sense Making and Paying Attention

Table 5.1 Comparison of Traditional and Contemporary Views of the Organization

	Traditional Organizational Paradigm	Contemporary Organizational Paradigm
Basic Assumption of Organizational Functioning	• Organizations are machinelike and predictable (based on Newtonian theory) • Organizations are stable and controllable • An understanding of the parts leads to an understanding of the whole • Cause and effect	• Organizations are holistic and the parts are interrelated and indivisible • Organizations are essentially unknowable and unpredictable • Organizations are similar to living systems, which are complex and adaptive • The sum of the whole is greater than the individual parts
Relationships	• Fragmentation • Specialization • Departmentalization	• Central to the working of the organizations • Diverse practitioners work together
Control	• Emphasis on planning, directing, controlling, and evaluating • Predictable outcomes	• Fosters creativity, risk taking • Unpredictable outcomes
Change	• Planned • Seeks simplicity and order • Change mandated from the top	• Evolutionary • Comfortable with experimentation and disruption • Change emerges from the bottom
Information	• Flows primarily downward with formal systems for upward communications	• Open, loose, diverse
Role of the Leader	• Decision maker	• Sense maker
Structure	• Hierarchical	• Microsystems • Semiautonomous work units

- Strategy 4: Taking Action: Small Steps, Multiple Steps
- Strategy 5: Letting Go: Accepting What You Cannot or Should Not Control
- Strategy 6: Having Fun!

At this point we want to stress that although your role changes from being in rigid control and the ultimate decision maker, this does not imply that you are to be inactive or passive. Your role is to be a transformational leader by setting high expectations, assuring that the job is done well, designing systems to bring out the best in the team and the individual staff members, resolving conflicts, and taking action when things are not going well. The end result is that everyone comes to work with joy and a passion for what they do.

Strategy 1: Fostering Relationships

The premier strategy suggested by complexity science is that clinical units (microsystems) must be designed to cultivate relationships among diverse individuals in the organization and to provide them with the information that they need. In our traditional organizational systems, characterized by a chain of command, departmentalization, and specialization among the clinical and administrative practitioners, relationships and information flow are hampered. McDaniel (1997) proposes that the key to successful leadership is developing and managing complex relationships among people who are diverse and significantly different from one another. This team of people should be supported in learning together, adapting to the environment and solving problems in an unpredictable and unknowable health care environment, allowing creativity and adaptability to emerge.

The role of the clinical leader is to design new formal and informal systems that put together diverse members of the multidisciplinary team from both within and outside your unit. Once these connections are made, information sharing should be loose and open with everyone having as much information as possible.

An example of making new connections recently happened as a result of a managerial workshop on change and complexity. The manager of the Emergency Department (ED) complained to the clinical manager of a psychiatric inpatient unit that they were not accepting patients quickly enough and backing up the ED. She assigned members of her staff to the ED for a day to follow their patients and work with an ED nurse. Likewise, some of the ED staff went to the inpatient unit for a day. From these new connections and information sharing emerged an understanding of the constraints and barriers in both systems and ideas from both staff for enhancing patient flow and admissions. From this example you can see that making connections does not depend on having meetings but results from working with one another, informal conversations at lunch, and informal hallway conversations, to name a few.

Table 5.2   Questions for Making Connections

- Who needs to connect with whom?
- Who outside of the unit needs to connect with people in the unit?
- How can I get the appropriate people involved?
- Who are the informal leaders and how should they relate?
- What information does the team need and how should they get that information?
- How should information flow?
- And continuously ask, who else?

Table 5.2 is a set of questions you might use to think through how to facilitate making connections in your organization. Although seemingly simple questions, they do structure your thinking so that you are inclusive.

Your role does not end with setting up the systems. You will need to be available to the staff as conflict is inevitable. Linda Rusch, the Vice President of Patient Care Services at Hunterdon Medical Center, who has embraced complexity science as a leadership approach (see Chapter 18), says:

"My job is to bring all the relationships together, and help people learn, like teaching conflict resolution. When people are afraid of hurting other people, they don't resolve conflicts and that's very dysfunctional. The relationship goes deeper and is more meaningful when you can resolve the conflict" (Regine, n.d.).

In every organization an informal network, frequently called the *shadow system* in complexity science lingo, exists and often works better than formal systems of meetings and councils. It is an example of complexity science in action and is also where creativity and innovation can occur. We suggest that you gain a better understanding of this system and use it for networking and to enhance information flow.

Strategy 2: Viewing the Organization Through the Lens of Complexity

Simply put, yet difficult to practice, the clinical leader needs to adopt a new view of the organization as complex, unpredictable, and uncontrollable. As we have seen, this is in direct conflict with how you have viewed your organization and your role in the past. Using the *lens of complexity* (Burns, 2001) can assist you in identifying and using the leadership strategies we are suggesting. You need to internalize a value that change can happen by letting things emerge, engage in risk taking, and allow people to be creative. This is difficult to accomplish when you and others have viewed the organization as machinelike.

Strategy 3: Sense Making and Paying Attention

Leading in complex organizations means helping the staff make sense of what is happening. It is answering the "why" question. You must understand this yourself by paying attention to the external and internal environment and asking "why?"

To see what is happening on your unit and in the organization, you have to be there, be seen, and be heard. This strategy, first identified in 1982 in the classic work by Peters and Waterman (p. 122), was called *management by wandering around*; it remains a viable and important strategy for the clinical manager today. Benefits of "wandering around" are:

- You can set expectations by finding people doing things right and providing positive feedback.
- You can communicate the vision and values informally.
- You can talk to and work with the "shadow system."
- You can identify problems.
- You can figure out what connections are being made and where they are not happening.

Strategy 4: Taking Action: Small Steps, Multiple Steps

The next strategy suggests that taking action in small, incremental steps is often better than complex planning. These actions are taken based on "good enough" plans having a few simple specifications as guidelines. This allows for better strategies and ways of doing things to emerge from many individuals. It also allows for small successes to happen that can build confidence, energize people for more change, and calm the doubters. Paradoxically, it also allows for failures to happen, but when they do they are small moments of learning rather than large setbacks. New actions and ideas emerge from the failures as well as from the successes.

The strategy of *taking multiple actions* deserves some attention and is a strategy popularized by looking at the organization through the lens of complexity science. This means implementing more than one action at a time for solving a problem or implementing a new direction or program. Although this can be at times confusing, and perhaps resource intensive, it also allows for the best solutions to emerge through the trial and error of several solutions. For example, you may want to set up a system to get more information from clients about their satisfaction with your services. You could start several initiatives at the same time such as focus groups that you lead, focus groups led by other staff or people outside your unit, written surveys, and informal rounds. Likewise, you could get information from families and physicians at the same time. By doing this you not only can potentially get richer information but you can determine which strategy is best and that you might use on a long-term basis.

Strategy 5: Letting Go: Accepting What You Cannot or Should Not Control

Morgan (n.d.) proposes that most people have about 15 percent control over their work situation. Organizationally imposed structures and systems over which you have no control make up the other 85 percent. Recognizing this and then deciding what you can influence helps you to spend your time in activities where you can be effective. Knowing this can help you be a successful leader as well as to avoid stress and burnout.

Learning to "let go" is another important lesson from complexity science. Davidhizar and Shearer (2002) suggest techniques to help you learn to let go:

- Avoid rushing in with personal interventions. You should first analyze the situation and decide if you personally need to take action or if you should serve in a consultative role.
- Do not react too early to an issue. When there is a problem, allow time for people to "cool off" and make sense of the issue so that it can be discussed calmly and you can all get more information to gain a better understanding.
- Build others' self-confidence so that they are comfortable in acting without your approval.
- Determine what you should say and when you should say it. Although we strongly believe that information should be shared broadly, there is a fine line between "telling people" what to do and why they should do it and letting them experience discovery.
- Talk last and practice active listening first; provide support rather than taking action on your own.

Strategy 6: Having Fun!

We think that complexity science frees you to experiment, allows you to be "out of control," unburdens you from bureaucracy, and thus allows you to have fun. The best contemporary prescription for having fun in the workplace appeared in the book *Fish!* (Lundin, Paul, & Christensen, 2000). We give the basic concepts of *Fish!* but strongly encourage you to read the original work. The *Fish!* philosophy came from the success of the Pike Place Fish Market in Seattle. The leaders of the fish market designed an organizational culture around four basic concepts:

- Play: Have fun at work by adopting a lighthearted, spontaneous approach to work.
- Be present: Be there for each other and for the client.

- Make their day: Perform small kindnesses and words for the client by going the extra mile.
- Choose your attitude: Come to work with a positive attitude; choose to love your work.

CHANGE

In the second half of this chapter, we review traditional change theory and integrate what we have learned about complexity science into a new change model using traditional aspects of change modified by complexity science. In other words, this is an example of "and/both" thinking. Both complexity science and traditional change theory can together inform you on how to handle the ever-present demands for change.

Traditional change theory models have a varying number of steps depending on the model's developer. But all basically have four distinct functions: assessing, setting objectives, implementing change, and evaluating. A distinctive characteristic of most change theories is the concept of resistance to change: people naturally resist change, and specific strategies can overcome this resistance. Although in our model we do consider how to analyze and deal with resistance to change, by using a complexity framework we believe there will be less resistance if the change is not imposed from the top down. Further, complexity science embraces resistance as often being positive; resistance challenges the processes, providing diversity of thoughts and opinions to assure that the best approaches are pursued. In our model the emphasis is on helping people to learn, grow, and adapt to internal and environmental factors so that they serve as architects of the change.

The Dimensions of Change

There are three dimensions of change: the *sources* from which it arises, the level of *complexity* of the change, and the multiple *demands* for change. When looking at organizational change from the perspective of a clinical leader, you are faced with demands for changes from several sources. These include:

- Changes suggested by staff and other stakeholders at the local level of your unit. These changes emerge from the clinical unit to improve client outcomes and system processes.
- Changes that you would like to see happen on your unit based on your personal scan of the internal and external environment.
- Changes that are imposed on you by the organization. Often these changes are imposed on the organization by regulators, payers, and societal values.

Changes can range from simple to complex. Another useful way to think about the dimensions of the changes that challenge you is to categorize them into first-order change and second-order change (Berguist, 1993). First-order change refers to small changes regarding some aspect of daily operations in which you do more or less of the same thing or do it in a slightly different way. For example, the use of a new flow sheet to document certain therapies would be a first-order change in which you do the same thing with a slight variation from the past. Second-order changes are major transformational changes of the systems in which you do things in significantly different ways. For instance, changing from a written system of order entry to computerized entry can significantly change the work of the unit.

And further complicating change is that you are usually dealing with more than one change demand at a time. This then means you need to think about and strategize how you will approach each change and manage your time.

A Change Model

The model below can be used as a framework for any changes you need to make, but should be modified depending on the source of the change and the complexity of the change.

The role of the clinical leader is to design an environment where people can learn, where change is embraced, and where creativity and innovation are fostered. This means that you must look inward first and reflect on your beliefs about change and the change process. For instance, you may or may not embrace an imposed organizational change, but it is your job to lead change nonetheless after raising objections and alternatives in an appropriate setting.

Our change model has six distinct functions (see Figure 5.1). We have purposely not numbered these functions because we do not believe that these happen in order or sequence; we present them in a circle in which the phases cycle back and return, at times gaining support and picking up speed.

- Creating dissatisfaction
- Forming a change team
- Developing and communicating a change vision
- Determining change strategies
- Taking action
- Evaluating outcomes

Creating Dissatisfaction

Because of your distinct position and responsibilities in the organization, as the clinical leader you are most likely the individual with the most information about the need for change in your unit due to demands from the external

Figure 5.1   A Change Model

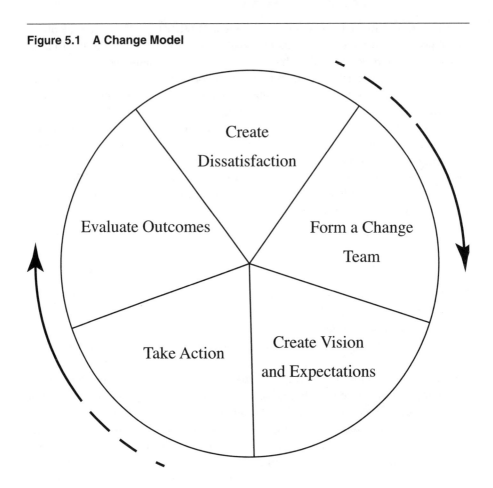

environment and those from inside the organization. The first step is to create urgency for the change and the rationale for the change. Although the term dissatisfaction has a negative connotation, we have chosen to use this term because it is important to understand that change does not happen unless people are dissatisfied with the status quo. Your job is to help people to become dissatisfied, understand why they are dissatisfied, explain the reasons for the change, create a vision that things will be better, and start taking action to improve outcomes and systems. Here are some strategies you can use:

- Set high expectations related to system processes and client outcomes.
- Provide data and information about the internal environment including its weaknesses, strategic initiatives, and competitors' threat.

- Make sure the staff understands the issues and trends in the external environment and the impact on their work.
- Measure performance of the unit and discuss areas needing improvement.
- Have staff interview dissatisfied patients and families.
- Have staff interact with the physicians and other stakeholders who are dissatisfied.
- Have honest discussion about what you see is needed.

Forming a Change Team

No matter the source or magnitude of the change, based on what we know about complexity science, you cannot demand and implement change by yourself. Further, the ultimate change will be better and more sustained if you make the connections among the people who need to be involved so that the final outcome is greater than the contribution any one person can make. In deciding who to put on your team, remember the fundamental principle of diversity and include key staff members, including all appropriate disciplines, all shifts, all levels of personnel, and informal leaders. Further, you need to assure that there is broad expertise in the group. Members need to be credible and able to build trust not only among themselves or the team, but they need to be seen as trustworthy by those affected by change. Once you form the team continue to ask the team and yourself, "Who else needs to be included?"

Developing and Communicating a Change Vision

Just as you have a broad overall vision for your unit, you should have a vision specific to the change initiative. The change vision will provide direction by clarifying the general direction you are headed, simplifying more detailed decisions as you move forward, and aligning the actions of the team. You can use Chapter 9 for developing and communicating the change vision.

Determining Change Strategies

Although we think complexity science can inform the change process in many ways, we also believe the traditional approach should be used to determine plans for change. Facilitating and restricting factors need to be assessed, written goals and plans are needed, responsibilities assigned, and timelines determined. Human nature and the busyness of each day will interfere with ultimate success if this step is not well thought out. However, complexity science suggests that doing this must happen quickly—weeks not months—and that there is an art to planning well, but not perfectly, looking for "good enough" so that actions can happen quickly.

Table 5.3   Assessing Facilitating and Restraining Factors

	Facilitating Factors	Strategies	Restraining Factors	Strategies
People				
Technology				
Values				
Structures				

The first step in our model is to assess the environment for its readiness for the change. In his classic work on change, Lewin (1947) proposed that there are both facilitators of change and barriers to change that must be assessed, understood, and appropriate strategies adopted to strengthen the facilitating factors and decrease the barriers. The facilitators and barriers can be people, technology, values, and structures. Table 5.3 can be used by the change team to analyze and discuss these factors and determine strategies for enhancing the facilitating factors and minimizing the barriers. Again we suggest that this exercise be undertaken in one or two meetings with the goal being to implement action quickly but reasonably.

After the assessment is completed, strategies for dealing with each factor can be determined. These strategies are derived from both what we now know about complexity science and the traditional paradigm:

People Strategies

- Cultivating an environment for inquiry
- Sharing information widely
- Providing connections and relationships among the staff
- Assuring wide participation of individuals
- Empowering the team and individuals to act
- Educating and developing staff as needed

Value Strategies

- Visioning
- Understanding and changing old habits
- Designing a climate for change in which risk taking is the norm and failures are acceptable

Technology

- Assessing resources and securing what is needed to make the change

Table 5.4   Planning Change Worksheet

Objective	Plan	Responsible Person	Timeline	Evaluation/ Outcomes

Structure/Systems

- Assessing these for function
- Making the changes needed

Next the team plans the change in some detail, but again looking for general guidelines, not letting the planning stand in the way of acting. The team can use Table 5.4 as a template for documenting goals, plans, timelines, the responsible parties for each plan, and how to evaluate success.

Taking Action

We suggest that you take small steps and multiple steps at the same time if appropriate to your needs. When there is a major, imposed transformational change this may not be possible, and you may have to take a major action all at once, such as when a new information system "goes live." But even then, most large changes occur in a step-wise fashion with one action building on the next.

The goal is to have a broad base of action, involving as many people as you can. Over time you can accelerate the pace of change as small changes emerge and you can build on them and learn what is not working as well.

Evaluating Outcomes

This step has its basis firmly in the old world paradigm where you measure success based on reaching goals that are measurable. You can use Table 5.5 as a template for thinking this through. Move the last column of Table 5.4 to the first column of this table and think about how you will measure each outcome.

We encourage you to measure with numbers and written surveys but also to use some qualitative measurements. One way to do this is to prepare a few

Table 5.5   Template for Measuring Change Outcomes

Outcome	Methods and Tools for Measuring	Responsibility	Timelines

broad questions and interview the staff, patients, and families affected by the change. For issues of patient satisfaction you can get much richer data by talking to patients than you can from the standard patient satisfaction surveys while providing meaningful involvement for the staff.

APPLICATION EXERCISES

1. Think about what relationships and connections currently occur on your unit. How can you foster more connections and information flow?
2. Who is the shadow system in your unit?
3. View the organization and your unit through the lens of complexity. Use Table 5.1.
4. "Wander around your unit" and learn three new things about the people or systems. Provide positive feedback to three people. How can you make this a routine?
5. Think about how the 15/85 rule applies to you. What strategies can you use to "let go"?
6. Think about a change that occurred as a result of small actions that grew into a change. What patterns and themes do you see in this example?
7. Use the change model to implement a small change on your unit and analyze what goes well and what does not.
8. Skip to Chapter 17 and read the chapter entitled "Complexity Science in Action."

REFERENCES

Anderson, R. A., Issel, L. M., & McDaniel, R. R. (2003). Nursing homes as complex adaptive systems. *Nursing Research, 52* (1), 12–21.

Berguist, W. (1993). *The modern organization: Mastering the art of irreversible change.* San Francisco: Jossey-Bass.

Burns, J. P. (2001). Complexity science and leadership in healthcare. *Journal of Nursing Administration, 31,* 474–482.

Davidhizar, R. & Shearer, R. (2002). Taking charge by "letting go." *Health Care Management, 20* (3), 33–37.

Lanza, M. L. (2000). Nonlinear dynamic: Chaos and catastrophe theory. *Journal of Nursing Care Quality, 15* (1), 55–65.

Lewin, K. (1947). Frontiers in group dynamics: Concepts, method, and reality in social science, social equilibrium, and social change. *Human Relations, 1* (1), 5–41.

Lundin, S. C., Paul, H., & Christensen, J. (2000). *Fish! A remarkable way to boost morale and improve results.* New York: Hyperion.

McDaniel, R. R. (1997). Strategic leadership: A view from quantum in chaos theories. *Healthcare Management Review, 22* (1), 21–37.

Peters, T. J., & Waterman, R. H. (1982). *In search of excellence: Lessons from America's best-run companies.* New York: Warner Communications.

Plsek, P. (2003, January 27–28). *Complexity and adoption of innovation in health care.* Paper presented at the meeting of the Accelerating Quality Improvement in Health Care: Strategies to Speed the Diffusion of Evidence-Based Innovations. Retrieved October 16, 2003, from http://www.aacn.nche.edu/Publications/White Papers/Plsek.pdf.

Regine, B. (n.d.). *The Hunterdon Medical Center: Critical mass and the emergence of the goddess.* Retrieved September 23, 2004, from http://www.plexusinstitute.org/services/stories/show.cfm?id=14.

Wheatley, M. J. (1994). *Leadership and the new science: Learning about organization from an orderly universe.* San Francisco: Berrett-Koehler Publishers.

Zimmerman, B., Lindberg, C., & Plsek, P. (n.d.). *A complexity science primer: What is complexity science and why should I learn about it?* Retrieved January 17, 2005, from Plexus Institute Web site: http://plexusinstitute.com/services/E-library/show.cfm?id=150.

CHAPTER 6

Managing Personal Resources: Time and Stress Management

Anne M. Barker

INTRODUCTION

As we saw in Chapter 3, Leadership IQ research found that effective leaders spend their time across the eight leadership roles; however, the most effective leaders spent the most significant amount of their time in the problem solver role, anticipating and actively seeking issues to be resolved before they become crises. The next most significant block of time was devoted to the other leader roles, with maintenance or routine administrative functions allocated the least amount of time (Murphy, 1996). Highly effective leaders retain their focus and spend their most precious resource—time—in the areas that will mobilize the team to achieve organizational goals. Unfortunately, many managers do not have an accurate picture of how they spend their time, and may be driven away from priority actions by bureaucratic demands. Excellent leaders exhibit strategies to accomplish the necessary administrative tasks without allowing them to compromise the key leadership roles and functions.

By completing the exercises and assessments in this chapter, you should gain a better understanding of your strengths and weaknesses regarding time and stress management. Once you have done this you can refocus your time to address the important work of leadership.

TIME MANAGEMENT

Time is one of the most precious resources that you have and one you can control. To be effective and efficient in your role as clinical leader, you need to manage your time so that you can spend your time in activities that move forward the vision, goals, and success of your clinical unit while at the same time gaining satisfaction and enjoyment in your role.

Benefits of Managing Your Time

The traditional view of time management is that time is a precious resource that must be managed. However, there is more to time management than only thinking of it as a resource. The most important benefits of time management are (Barker, 1992, pp. 189–190):

- Having clarity of mind. When you manage your time well, you can have a clear, calm mind when confronted with the multiple demands of your role. In the confusion and disorder of daily activities and crises, you still must pay attention to the most important aspects of your job—designing and maintaining a satisfying work environment that retains staff and results in positive client outcomes. If you are struggling to accomplish daily tasks and to keep on top of your workload, you will not have the peace of mind to reflect on your own practice, be there for others, and act proactively.
- Conserving personal energy. You have a limited amount of energy to use for the achievement of your professional and personal goals, no matter how vigorous and energetic you are. Another goal of managing your time is to minimize the number of demands on you at any one time to assure that you have adequate energy at all times.
- Nonverbal messaging about significance. How you spend your time sends a message to others about what you think is important and what you do not think is important. It is in essence "walking the talk" or spending time on important activities. When you view time management from this perspective, you can see that it is, in fact, another strategy for building trust.
- Contributing to feelings of well-being and happiness. When you manage your time, you will feel more in control of your life, less stressed, and be less likely to experience burnout. In fact, personal success can be

measured by how you spend your time and if you are spending it on activities that bring meaning, satisfaction, and joy to your life.

Consequences of Poor Time Management

The consequences of not managing your time well include:

- Being unable to manage yourself. First of all, managing your time means managing yourself. As a leader, if you cannot manage yourself, it seems obvious that you will not be able to manage and lead others.
- Negatively impacting others. Your entire clinical unit, and even your department, can be negatively affected if you do not complete your work and projects on time. Other people often rely on your input and work to complete their work. It is simply unfair to others not to be timely in submission of your work. Further, the staff on your unit can feel off balance when there are issues that remain unresolved (Barker, 1992, pp. 190–191).
- Promoting distrust. When you do not have the time to follow through on decisions and actions that you have promised, people will not trust you.

Time Management: Self-Assessment

In this section we present two approaches to assess your time management skills. We strongly encourage you to complete these activities if you are experiencing any one of the following:

- Regularly exceeding the number of required hours spent on the job
- Regularly taking work home and working in the evenings and on weekends
- Feeling resentful about the amount of time that you must devote to your position
- Not having clarity of mind
- Constantly feeling rushed and out of control
- Feeling that you do not have time to embrace the leadership strategies discussed in this book
- Not having time for personal reflection and growth

The good news is that you can gain control over your time. Time management experts believe that people waste on average two to three hours per day as a result of ineffective use of time (Davenport, 1982, p. 52). By assessing how you use your time and adopting the suggested techniques, you should be able to capture some of this wasted time for more meaningful and important activities.

However, we make this statement with one caveat. There are organizational cultures that continuously place unrealistic demands upon the managers in the organization and/or continuously have last-minute, "urgent" requests for reports, attending meetings, and so forth. You will need to evaluate for yourself if you are working in such a culture, or are your own time management issues the problem. If your situation is partially or totally an organizational culture issue, you can ask for your mentor's help in learning to negotiate how to say "no" and accepting the fact that this is the culture and you may have little influence. Be careful, however, not to "blame" the culture as you self-reflect. One of the best ways to do this is to talk with your peers about time management.

We suggest you engage in two activities to assess your time management strengths and weaknesses. The first is to do a brief self-assessment (see Table 6.1). Once you have completed the assessment pay particular attention in your reading about those areas in which you scored a 3 or less.

The second way to assess how you are spending your time is to keep a time log for at least one week. This is a more detailed assessment but is well worth the effort. It is best to keep a time management log for both organizational time and personal time, since the goal is for you to have a balance between both aspects of your life.

Table 6.2 is a time log format that you can use for completing this activity. In column 1 indicate the time you begin and end an activity. You should make an entry every time you switch activities. In column 2 state what the activity is and who is involved in this activity with you. In column 3 you should state the purpose of the activity. (This is to help you see if you are spending your time in activities that you deem important for the leadership of your unit versus mundane and even unmeaningful tasks.) Use column 4 to indicate your energy level: L for low, M for medium, and H for high. (The purpose of reflecting on your energy level is to analyze if you are doing your most important work when your energy level is highest.) In column 5 note if you are interrupted while you are completing the activity and make notes about who interrupted and the reason for it. You can rate each interruption as very important (VI), important (I), or little importance (LI). In the last column, make notes about the effectiveness of how you spent your time as soon as possible after the event or at the end of the day. Questions that you might ask yourself when completing this column are:

- Was this activity directly related to the mission of the unit, the satisfaction of the staff, or assuring positive patient outcomes?

Table 6.1   Assessment Tool for Time Management

Use the following scoring system for each answer below.
Place an X in the appropriate column.
1 = Never
2 = Rarely
3 = Occasionally
4 = Usually
5 = Always

	1	2	3	4	5
I feel calm and in control of my time.					
I am aware of fluctuations in my energy level and perform my most challenging tasks when my energy level is at its highest.					
I spend the majority of my time in meaningful work that contributes to the positive work on my clinical unit.					
I spend the majority of my time in activities that I find satisfying.					
I complete my paperwork and projects on time.					
I follow through on promises I make to my staff, boss, and others.					
I have written daily goals.					
I delegate tasks to others in my clinical unit.					
I assess tasks for their importance and their urgency.					
I keep a "to do" list and schedule time to complete the tasks on the list.					
I set aside time each week to complete paperwork and other tasks.					
I am able to control interruptions.					
I embrace the philosophy "do today instead of putting off until tomorrow."					
I set aside time each day for planning.					
I have written long term goals.					

Table 6.2   Time Management Log

Time	Activity/ People	Purpose	Energy Level	Interruptions	Effectiveness of the Time Spent

- Could the task have been done in a better way or delegated?
- Did I spend too much or not enough time on the activity? Was I able to complete the task?
- Was the task performed at the right time in relationship to my energy level?

At the end of the week perform an analysis of the entire week as a whole. Besides the questions above, other questions to ask yourself are:

- What percentage of my time is spent in work, family, home, social, spiritual, and physical activities? Do I have the balance of these that I want?
- What percentage of my time do I spend in activities that are important or urgent?
- Who am I spending time with and are they the most appropriate people to help me reach my goals and those of the clinical unit?
- What are my main interruptions? Assess the percentage of time they fall into each of the categories: very important, important, little importance? How can I decrease the number of unimportant interruptions?
- What are my biggest time wasters?
- Are there any activities I can reduce or eliminate?
- Is there anything I can delegate to others or simplify?
- Can I save time by grouping related tasks?
- Were there any tasks that I had put off and then was under pressure to complete?

If you find this activity useful, we suggest that you complete it annually or more often if and when you need a "time management" tune-up. This will help you see where you have improved and what else you can do in the future. Time management is not easy and there are times when you will experience setbacks and days when you will not feel you have managed your time well; this is perfectly normal. It takes constant care and attention to be a good manager of your time.

Strategies for Managing Your Time

In this section we present strategies to help you manage your time. Based on your self-assessment and the findings from your time management log, choose several strategies that you think will provide the most leverage in managing your time. The conventional wisdom is that it is using these strategies collectively, not in isolation of one another, that will give you the best results (Seaward, 2004).

Goal Setting and Planning

Most time management experts agree that goal setting and planning are the premier time management strategies. In this section we suggest ways to plan for goal achievement.

Your goals are derived from three sources. First are the daily, regularly changing tasks that you need to complete such as paperwork, committee assignments, performance appraisals, budget development and review, to name a few. Second, there are goals that are derived from the organization and unit vision and strategic plans (see Chapter 9). Finally, there are goals for your personal development and growth (see Chapter 4). All three need to be worked on at the same time. The techniques suggested below can be applied to all your goals no matter their purpose.

First, write down your goals. Once you have written goals, you should carry them with you in a day planner or personal digital assistant (PDA), a handheld computer. You should do two complementary things with these written goals. First, look at your goals daily to keep them fresh in your mind. By doing this, you will be more sensitive to opportunities that will help you reach your goals.

At the beginning of each day you should have a list of activities to accomplish that day to move you toward your written goals. This should be a list of activities that help you to accomplish routine and required tasks, the vision and strategic plan, and your own personal development. In this way you can assure you have a balance between working on both your short-term and long-term goals.

It is not easy to set realistic daily goals; at first you will probably plan more than you can accomplish, but as time progresses you will get better at doing this. Most important, do not get frustrated if you don't accomplish every task every day. In fact, one time management principle suggests that a task will consume the time you have allotted for it. Therefore, planning an aggressive schedule is a good strategy as long as you do not get frustrated that you did not accomplish everything you set out to do.

Barker (1992) suggests a number of guidelines to follow when setting goals:

- Goals should include all aspects of your life, including your work, family, social, financial, spiritual, physical, and psychological areas.
- Goals should be measurable, achievable yet challenging.

- In determining realistic goals consider organizational constraints, resources, and your personal strengths and skills.
- Set time frames for goal completion that are realistic but do not allow for procrastination. You can reassess timelines and set new deadlines and add new goals or drop old ones when appropriate.
- Reward yourself upon completion of goals.
- Pursue your goals with enthusiasm, even when you are not feeling enthusiastic.

Scheduling

You should have a calendar/day planner/PDA in which to schedule meetings, make plans for time to accomplish your tasks, keep your goals, and have an ongoing "to do" list. Each day when you review your goals you should also review your schedule and block in time to accomplish daily tasks and work on long-term goals.

You need to see not only what the schedule for each day is, but you need a broader view of the week and month. You can put deadlines into the planner and block out times to work on projects or paperwork to accomplish them in a timely manner. There are two benefits to doing this: it assures you have a plan to get your work completed on time and you do not have to worry needlessly about when and how you are going to accomplish it.

Prioritizing Tasks: Urgent Versus Important

A useful way of prioritizing your daily list of goals and tasks is to consider whether the task is important or not important and if it is urgent or not urgent. You can use Figure 6.1 to develop your own template to assess importance and urgency of tasks and then prioritize your daily activities accordingly. On the vertical axis is a rating of urgency from low to high, and on the horizontal axis is a rating of importance from low to high. Place each activity in one of the four quadrants. First complete the tasks in quadrant I, those that rate a high urgent and high importance score. Next complete the activities in quadrant II, which are high importance and low urgency. Next complete the activities in quadrant III, which are low importance and high urgency. And finally complete those tasks low in urgency and importance. The grid prioritizes your tasks by importance first and urgency second.

Another complementary way to prioritize daily activities is to understand the Pareto principle, also known as the 80/20 rule. This principle suggests that 80 percent of positive, satisfying outcomes are a result of just 20 percent of the time that you spend. Or in other words, paying attention to your important tasks will give you 80 percent of the results. You can use this principle when assigning

Figure 6.1   Assessing Tasks for Importance and Urgency

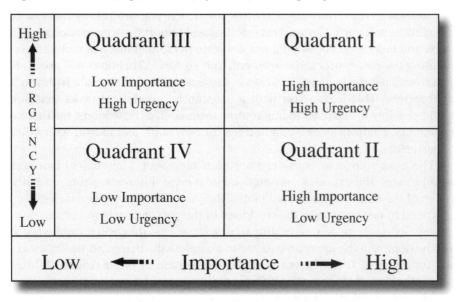

importance to each task in the grid. You can also see by applying this principle that minor changes to your time management skills can produce dramatic results.

Delegation

The majority of your time should be spent moving forward the vision and mission of your clinical unit. To do this, you need to delegate tasks to other people on the unit. However, many clinical managers have difficulty delegating due to attitudes and values that they hold. Before you can successfully delegate to others, you need to think about your attitude and values about delegating. Here are some useful ways to think positively about delegation:

- Delegation is a trust-building activity.
- Delegation builds the confidence and self-esteem of others.
- Delegation unburdens you from routine, mundane tasks to provide you the time for important activities and relationship building.
- Delegation helps others to grow, learn, and become leaders as they see more of the "big picture."
- Delegation is an important tool in succession planning.
- Delegation can match the right person with the right expertise to the right job.

The process of delegation involves looking at the task(s) you plan to delegate and the people to whom you will delegate. Some tasks you should not delegate. These include activities for which you are the figurehead of the clinical unit such as award ceremonies and important organizational functions and meetings. You should not delegate personnel matters including rewarding people, conflict management, and so forth. This does not preclude you from having other staff involved in these activities side by side with you if appropriate. This leaves you with a substantial number of tasks that you might possibly delegate including routine tasks such as scheduling, making assignments, chairing search committees for new staff, and liaison with other departments.

The next step is to consider your staff members. The clinical manager should judge the expertise, strengths, knowledge, interests, skills, and attitudes of the staff. These should match the job to be done. When delegating, you need to be sensitive to the workload of the person to whom you are delegating. Giving the person the ability to negotiate what they will do and when it will be done and the appropriate time to complete the delegated task is essential for success. It may mean relieving the person of other responsibilities during the time that the task is being completed.

The process that you use to delegate is important. First, the person needs to understand the importance of the task, why it is being delegated, and what are the requirements and guidelines. You will need to give appropriate information and provide the resources such as time, space, and money to complete the task. You should set dates for task completion and periodic evaluation if the task extends over a long time period. As difficult as this may be for you, you must understand that the results of the assignment are more important than the means by which the person completes them, as long as he or she completes the task consistent with the unit mission and working with others in a positive manner.

Throughout the process of task completion, you must be available to give the person advice, support, and guidance. Once the task is completed an appropriate reward needs to be given. The person should always be given the recognition and credit for the task both privately and in public.

Allowing Yourself Private Time

An oft-spoken value for which managers take great pride is having an open-door policy. There is a difference between having an open-door policy and having your door open all the time. One of the most effective time management strategies is to schedule and set aside time every week to close your door and to get required paperwork and tasks completed. We suggest you review your calendar and find a time when you do not have meetings and book in private time for two to four hours per week in one to two blocks of time for the next six months.

Of course, you cannot just suddenly close your door without explaining to the staff what you are doing and why. On the other hand, others need to respect your time so that you can accomplish the many demands that you have. One of the authors has a system that she uses to communicate availability:

- A closed door means, "Please do not bother me unless it's an emergency or crisis."
- A half-open door means, "I am doing an important task, would prefer not to be interrupted, but come in if you need to see me now and if it cannot wait until later."
- An open door means "Come on in!"

Controlling Interruptions

On average, we experience one interruption every 8 minutes or approximately seven per hour. In an eight-hour day, that totals around 50–60 interruptions in the day. The average interruption takes approximately 5 minutes. If you have 50 interruptions in the day and each takes 5 minutes, that totals 250 minutes, or 50 percent of the workday. Moreover, most people will discover that only about 20 percent of their interruptions are very important or important. Thus, if you experience 250 minutes of interruptions in your day and 80 percent have little value, then three hours per day are being consumed by interruptions that are not worthy of your time (Wetmore, 1999).

Looking at this math, you can easily see how you can capture time to devote to important leadership strategies. Go back over your time log and try to identify patterns in your interruptions, the time you spend dealing with them, and if there are people who tend to take more of your time than others. After this analysis you can then set some strategies to decrease your interruptions. For example, if one person interrupts you more than others, it might mean you need to schedule time with this person periodically and ask them to have a list of items to discuss with you rather than ask for your time "on the fly."

Procrastination and Perfectionism

Procrastination, putting off what you need to do until the last minute, is often referred to as "putting off until tomorrow what I should have done today." Procrastination can take several forms including knowingly doing something other than what needs to be done, starting to work on a project then stopping work on it only to have to complete it at the last minute, or doing less difficult tasks rather than the required one (Seaward, 2004, pp. 303–304). Being aware of your tendency toward procrastination is important in your understanding of your time management skills and in the strategies you adapt. Scheduling, maintaining "to do" lists, and adhering to them can help you break this habit.

A different but parallel problem is being a perfectionist. Perfectionists generally get caught up in the details and never see the whole picture; thus they waste time (Seaward, 2004, p. 304). Further, believing that you should and can be perfect is detrimental to your self-esteem. No one can be perfect. When you hold yourself up to a standard of perfection and you do not meet this standard, you then feel as if you failed. Recognizing your tendency to want to be perfect and moderating it is important not only to time management but also to self-esteem.

One way to reduce your need to be perfect is to consider what is "good enough." To do this, you make a judgment about the level of perfection/accuracy required for the specific task.

Managing Communications

Reading and responding to e-mail can consume a large portion of your time. Here are several hints for making the task more meaningful and less time consuming:

- Read your e-mail at least one to two times per day depending on your schedule and the volume you receive.
- Set up folders for your e-mails from important people, about meetings, or tasks to be done.
- Keep your inbox uncluttered by reading and responding to messages, then moving those e-mails to an appropriate folder if you need to keep them for the future. Otherwise, immediately delete e-mails that do not need to be saved.
- Respond immediately to e-mails that need short responses and then move the e-mails or delete them.
- Read e-mails that are marked as urgent first.
- Sort your e-mail by sender and read e-mails from your boss, your staff, and other important contacts in the organization next.
- If an e-mail cannot be responded to quickly and you do not have time to answer it, schedule time for a response at a later time. Print the e-mail as a reminder to follow up.

Managing phone calls is another important time management technique. Phone conversations can be much more pertinent and personal than e-mails, but learn to keep your calls to fewer than 5 minutes. The downside of phone calls is that you often find yourself playing "phone tag," which can be a time waster. When you leave a person voice mail, specify a good time for the person to return your call so that you increase the possibility of being available when the person calls.

If you have a support person who answers the phone, you should give instructions for how to handle your phone calls. Whoever is taking calls should be able to screen calls and refer the caller to the appropriate person if it is not you. You can ask the support person to find out when a convenient time is to return the call or even to schedule a phone appointment if the person keeps your calendar. You can also instruct on how to communicate your availability. For example, saying that "she is not on the unit" is a different message than saying "she is at x meeting and I expect her back in an hour."

STRESS MANAGEMENT

As health care professionals you should already be familiar with the physiology of stress and stress-related diseases. Stress management is a life skill and although important to your success as a clinical manager, much stress management occurs outside the workplace. No doubt you already use many different techniques to reduce your stress. In this section we look briefly at occupational stressors and provide some stress management techniques.

Occupational Stress

The National Safety Council (Seaward, 1994) lists many causes of job stress. How someone experiences and reacts to these stressors varies from person to person. Table 6.3 can be used as you assess job-related stress based on the reasons identified by the National Safety Council. After you complete the assessment, look closely at items that you rated 3 or more before you read the next section.

A Stress Management Model

People have many ways of dealing with stress. As you read this section, note the techniques that appeal to you. Using a mix of techniques can help you be more effective in dealing with stress. These techniques fall into three categories: altering behaviors to deal more effectively with stress, avoiding stress, or accepting stress (Tubesing & Tubesing, 1983). You may want to select at least one strategy from each category as a beginning point. Some of the techniques require behavioral approaches to managing stress while others require a change of thinking.

Table 6.3   Assessment Tool for Occupational Stress

Use the following scoring system for each answer below. Place an X in the appropriate column. 1 = Never 2 = Rarely 3 = Occasionally 4 = Usually 5 = Always					
	1	**2**	**3**	**4**	**5**
I have too much responsibility with little or no authority.					
The organization sets unrealistic expectations and deadlines that I am unable to meet.					
I do not feel adequately trained for my position.					
I do not feel appreciated.					
I am not able to voice concerns.					
I have too much to do with too few resources.					
I lack a clear understanding of what is expected of me.					
I have a difficult time keeping pace with technology.					
The physical environment in which I work has poor lighting, a lot of noise, and poor ventilation.					
There is the possibility of workplace violence.					
People in the organization have experienced sexual harassment and racial discrimination.					
The organization has recently downsized or restructured.					
Creativity and autonomy are not valued.					

The purpose of stress management is to adopt coping skills. *Coping* is defined as the process of managing demands that are perceived by the person as demanding or exceeding the individual's resources. The purpose of coping skills can be to reduce the harmful effects of the stressor, to be able to better tolerate or adjust to negative events, to maintain a positive self-image, and to keep emotional equilibrium while maintaining satisfying relationships with others (Lazarus, 1999).

Altering Techniques

Many stressors cannot be eliminated, but you can adopt techniques to alter how you deal with stress. These include:

- Problem solving
- Communication
- Making sure you have the right information
- Time management, priority setting, and planning
- Conflict management (Tubesing & Tubesing, 1983; Seaward, 2004)

Avoidance Techniques

A second set of strategies to deal with stress suggests that you avoid stress, rather than alter your reactions to it as discussed above. These strategies include:

- Using an assertive communications style
- Saying no and walking away
- Letting go
- Delegating tasks
- Being aware of your personal limitations and energy (Tubesing & Tubesing, 1983)

Acceptance Techniques

These acceptance techniques fall into two different categories. The first are techniques to build up your resistance to stress, and the second are cognitive approaches to change your perception of the stress.

Building Resistance to Stress. These techniques are probably most familiar to you as stress management techniques. They include such things as diaphragmatic breathing, meditation, yoga, music, massage, progressive muscular relaxation, nutrition, physical exercise, engaging in creative activities or hobbies, humor, and prayer.

Changing Perceptions of Stress. A second set of techniques are cognitive ones that help you deal more effectively with stress by changing your perceptions of both yourself and your reactions to stress. This set of techniques includes:

- Being optimistic and positive, rather than negative
- Using visualization and affirmation including positive self-talk
- Journal writing for self-expression and self-awareness
- Practicing forgiveness (Tubesing & Tubesing, 1983; Seaward, 2004)

APPLICATION EXERCISES

1. After reading the chapter, completing the assessments, and reviewing the strategies, add time management and stress management goals to your professional development plan (see Chapter 4).
2. Review your time log and time/stress management goals with your mentor.
3. Review the information regarding stress management, realistically assess how much stress you are experiencing, and choose several strategies to help you cope with stress. Use the Internet to do a search on the techniques you select.

REFERENCES

Barker, A. M. (1992). *Transformational nursing leadership: A vision for the future.* New York: National League for Nursing.

Davenport, R. (1982). *Making time, making money: A step by step process for setting your goals and achieving success.* New York: St. Martin's Press.

Lazarus, R. (1999). *Stress and emotion: A new synthesis.* New York: Springer Publishing Company.

Murphy, E. C. (1996). *Leadership IQ.* New York: John Wiley & Sons.

Seaward, B. L. (1994). *National Safety Council's stress management.* Sudbury, MA: Jones and Bartlett Publishers.

Seaward, B. L. (2004). *Managing stress: Principles and strategies for health and well-being* (4th ed.). Sudbury, MA: Jones and Bartlett Publishers.

Tubesing, N., & Tubesing, D. (1983). *Structured exercises in stress management.* Duluth, MN: Whole Person Press.

Wetmore, D. E. (1999). *The big hole in your day.* Retrieved February 15, 2005, from http://www.balancetime.com/articles/hole_in_your_day.htm.

Part Two

Part Two

CHAPTER 7

Leadership Competencies for Clinical Managers

Dori Taylor Sullivan

--------- CHAPTER QUESTIONS ---------

1. What are competencies?
2. How are competencies useful in the context of leadership practice and development for clinical managers?
3. Is there a set of recognized, common leadership competencies?
4. How do leadership competencies relate to the theories or lenses for viewing situations that clinical managers typically encounter?

INTRODUCTION

Our model of Multi-dimensional Leadership provides lenses or theories through which the role of the clinical manager can be viewed to enhance performance. In this section of the book, we move on to describing the nature of the clinical manager role, or what activities and responsibilities people in this role perform. The clinical manager role has evolved and changed in response to the dramatic and continuing modifications to the health care environment in which we practice.

This chapter will provide a summary of early definitions of the manager role, and then update you with detailed information regarding current thinking and research on what clinical leaders need to do in today's health care environment. Based on prior work and our analysis and experience, we propose seven competencies that clinical leaders should focus on to be effective in their role. Each of these competencies are defined and subsequent chapters provide in-depth information to assist you in enhancing your skills related to each one.

Defining Competencies

The term *competencies* is derived from *competence* or *competency*, commonly defined as the ability to do something successfully. We use the word competencies when describing the actions or behaviors expected from a person occupying a certain role successfully, in this case that of clinical leader. While there are many complex definitions of what competencies are, the simplest and most direct is that *competencies are what you can do with what you know*!

This definition implies that it is not enough to cognitively understand things, but rather the use of the necessary knowledge, skills, and attitudes in actual leadership practice is what counts. You may be thinking at this point of frequently overheard comments about people who may know a lot but cannot accomplish much or individuals who have not had formal education or training but repeatedly achieve more than others in leadership roles. This goes to the heart of why thinking about competencies is so valuable.

Knowledge is the intellectual information that you possess from whatever formal or informal sources accessed. Skills relate to specific tasks that must be performed in a given role, for example, the preparation of a budget in spreadsheet format. Attitudes are your general opinion or sense of something or a predisposition toward certain actions. Most attitudes are derived from your values regarding the item or behavior creating the reaction. If you have a positive attitude regarding the need to help those less fortunate, you might be expected to support or participate in volunteer activities with that goal.

Translating the necessary knowledge, skills, and attitudes into action is what creates competency. Since few if any roles have only one responsibility, the plural term *competencies* speaks to what individuals must be able to do in a given role to be effective and successful.

COMPETENCIES IN THE EDUCATION AND PRACTICE OF CLINICAL LEADERS

Competencies provide a wonderful framework for the education and practice of clinical leaders. The creation of a set of agreed upon competencies provides a language to describe specific behaviors, actions, or accountabilities that those in clinical leader roles must accept and perform. The knowledge, skills, and attitudes required to be a successful clinical leader may be obtained in many different ways, and diversity of education and experience is to be encouraged. However, it does all come down to being able to do the job and do it well—and that is where the competencies provide the necessary specifics.

Having established competencies for the clinical leader, or any other role under consideration, promotes:

- Consistency in leadership behavior and expectations
- A template for evaluating clinical leaders
- An approach to leadership development in new or weaker competencies in the workplace
- An organizing framework for collegiate programs in health care leadership and management majors

In the following section we briefly review the extensive work done over the last 40 or 50 years in relationship to management and leadership roles and competencies. We end with the proposed clinical leader competencies for the 21st century, which are used to organize the remainder of Part Two of this book.

Defining What Leaders and Managers Should Do

Organizational behavior experts have long been fascinated with trying to figure out exactly what leaders and managers should do to be most effective. A number of prominent authors have created, researched, and used various ways to organize our thinking about successful leadership. One approach uses a more conceptual model, identifying in general terms what types of activities leaders should enact, for example, decision making. The other major approach tends to focus on specific responsibilities or expectations for leaders within the context of current business and operational priorities such as establishing shared governance. Not surprisingly, the first approach tends to be somewhat timeless, while the second changes and evolves as new information about organizations and the role of managers emerges.

The next sections provide an overview of the most well-known writings on the topic of leadership or management roles, classic and contemporary, to provide a foundation for understanding the proposed clinical leader competencies for the 21st century.

Early Descriptions of Leader and Manager Roles

Management may be defined as "the art of getting things done, with emphasis upon processes and methods for insuring incisive action . . . and securing concerted action by groups of [men]" (Simon, 1976). Based on this definition, a manager is responsible for the processes by which organizational goals are achieved through the effective use of resources and the work of others when functioning in an assigned official position.

Leadership is often defined as "the ability of one person to influence another to act in a way desired by the first . . ." and "the influential increment over and above mechanical compliance with a routine directive of an organization [manager]." (Katz & Kahn, 1978.) This view of leadership implies that others wish to follow and broadens leadership outside of organizationally appointed management positions.

In his classic article on managers and leaders, Zaleznik (1977) and Bennis and Nanus (1985, 1987) asserted that managers and leaders are very different kinds of people who differ in motivation, personal history, and in how they think and act. Table 7.1 lists recently published differences between management and leadership (Marriner-Tomey, 2004, p. 169; Bennis and Nanus, 1985, 1997). While these postulations appeal to our sense of logic, the distinction between managers and leaders becomes cloudy as the concept of managerial effectiveness is explored, since most organizations achieve enhanced outcomes when managers exhibit leadership qualities in addition to competence in defined managerial processes. Despite the distinction that may, and perhaps should, be made between management and leadership, numerous articles and authors (including us) use the terms interchangeably.

Mintzberg's Managerial Roles

Three prominent experts in management and organizational behavior published significant works related to the roles of leaders and managers in the 1970s: Mintzberg, Katz, and Schein. Even today these conceptualizations serve as the foundation for most contemporary recommendations on leader

Table 7.1   Differences in Management Versus Leadership

	Leadership	Management
Motto	Do the right things	Do things right
Challenge	Change	Continuity
Focus	Purposes	Structure and procedures
Time Frame	Future	Present
Methods	Strategies	Schedules
Questions	Why?	Who, what, when, where, and how?
Outcomes	Journeys	Destinations
Human	Potential	Performance

(Tomey, 2004; Bennis & Nanus, 1985, 1997)

competencies. So, to familiarize you with these important contributions, a brief review of each one is included below.

Mintzberg (1973) defined a manager as the person in charge of an organization or subunit with formal authority that leads to interpersonal relations that provide information for decision making. He then proposed 10 roles for managers organized into three categories called interpersonal roles, informational roles, and decisional roles.

The three manager roles in the interpersonal cluster are figurehead, leader, and liaison. The figurehead role relates to ceremonial and formal representation of the organization or subunit. The leader role encompasses many of the responsibilities usually associated with managers like establishing organizational structure and responsibility for the work of others and outcomes. The liaison role recognizes the manager's need to link with others outside the vertical chain of command, such as peers from other departments, customers, and business associates. The interpersonal roles clearly speak to the importance of the manager's people skills in a variety of domains.

The informational roles include monitor, disseminator, and spokesperson. The manager is said to emerge as the "nerve center" of the organizational unit, with the responsibility and positioning to gather and use important information from a multitude of sources to further the work of the unit and its members. The monitor role refers to information gathering, especially related to environmental factors and intra-unit communications. The disseminator role reasonably follows with its focus on assuring that information is relayed in a timely manner to those who need it. The spokesperson role relates to the manager formally representing the unit or its work to other internal and external people of influence. For example, keeping information flowing to those above the manager in the organizational structure is as valid a spokesperson role as is presenting to an outside audience.

Finally, the decisional roles consist of entrepreneur, disturbance handler, resource allocator, and negotiator. The prior two categories note the importance of relating well to people to acquire and dispense the information necessary to run the organizational unit. The decisional roles might be seen as the heart of the manager role because it is here that managers put this information to use to set direction, strategy, and achieve desired outcomes. The entrepreneur fosters the successful performance of the unit through matching unit functions to changing environments and needs, thus improving its processes and outcomes. The disturbance handler role, in contrast to the entrepreneur, must deal effectively with conflicts or threats as they arise. A disturbance is defined as a situation that creates pressure for the manager to respond or that will negatively influence the work and/or members of the unit.

The resource allocator is the tangible expression of the manager's priorities for the unit and may also include changes to the unit's organizational structure, roles, and processes. One of the most important decisions managers make is about allocating their own time and energy. The negotiator role suggests the need to resolve situations in "real time" and falls largely to managers because of their broad information scope and strategic abilities.

Mintzberg further explains that each of these 10 roles contributes to integrated job performance; that is, no one role can be removed without affecting the manager's ability to do the others. In a later work Mintzberg concludes: "This description of managerial work should prove more important to managers than any prescription they might derive from it . . . *Managers' effectiveness is significantly influenced by their insight into their own work*" (Mintzberg, 1990, p. 13).

Katz's Skills of an Effective Administrator

Katz (1974) sought to describe the skills needed to be an effective administrator. He suggested that three key areas are necessary for administrator success: conceptual skill, technical or analytic ability, and interpersonal or human relations skills. Conceptual skill relates to being able to see the bigger picture and organize one's thinking in a logical and related manner. It has been said that nothing can be accomplished that the leader has not envisioned. Whether you agree with that statement in total, it does seem to be true that this type of skill and thinking is necessary in managerial roles. The second category relates to the ability to systematically use information to analyze and understand situations that call for action or decision making. Last, the interpersonal skills described by Katz are very similar to those described in Mintzberg's model. An additional contribution of Katz is his observation that depending upon a manager's level in an organization, the three categories are needed in varying degrees, with senior leaders having the most need for conceptual skills with less need for technical skills.

Schein (1975), writing around the same time as Katz, thought managers need analytic and interpersonal skills; he also spoke to a dimension he labeled emotional toughness or sufficient ego strength to deal with the many challenges

---

Table 7.2   Summary of Classic Leader and Manager Role Categories

Mintzberg (1973)	Katz (1974) & Schein (1975)
Interpersonal	Interpersonal
Informational	Analytical/technical
Decisional	Conceptual
	Emotional toughness

faced by a manager. Taken together, these four skill sets (conceptual, technical/analytical, human relations, and emotional toughness) provide an alternative way to consider the skills needed in the manager role. Table 7.2 lists the manager roles proposed by Mintzberg, Katz, and Schein.

SURVEY OF CONTEMPORARY STUDIES ON LEADERSHIP COMPETENCIES

Numerous authors over the years have expanded on the work of Mintzberg, Katz, and Schein, validating many of the previously discussed concepts related to manager and leader roles. A review of more recent works related to health care leadership can provide a perspective on current thinking related to leadership competencies. Today's literature tends to deal with competencies more than roles.

Clinical Leader Competency Schemas

Since the late 1990s several authors have published articles proposing systems or schemas of health care leadership competencies. Competencies proposed by Perra (2001), Contino (2004), and Longest (2001) are compared in Table 7.3.

Perra (2001) suggested that effective leadership was critical to achieving quality outcomes in health care. She specifically referenced the nurse executive and manager charge to create a workforce that provides quality care in a creative and cost-effective manner. Perra proposed the integrated leadership practice model as a way to achieve these results. The model says the stated integrated leadership activities lead to staff participation and professional care that result in staff and customer satisfaction, which together define organizational

---

Table 7.3   Comparison of Contemporary Theories of Leadership Competencies

Perra (2001)	Contino (2004)	Longest (1998)
Self-knowledge, respect, trust, integrity, shared vision, participation, learning, communication, and change facilitator	Organizational management skills, communication skills, data/operational analysis and strategic planning skills, and creation/visionary skills	Conceptual, technical, management/clinical, interpersonal/collaboration, political, commercial, and governance

productivity. The integrated leadership characteristics and activities are self-knowledge, respect, trust, integrity, shared vision, participation, learning, communication, and change facilitator.

Similarly, Contino (2004) also proposed leadership competencies, defined as knowledge, skills, and aptitudes, that nurses need to lead organizations effectively. Her model of nurse leader competencies has four major categories: organizational management skills, communication skills, data/operational analysis and strategic planning skills, and creation/visionary skills.

In a popular 1998 article Longest described the leadership competencies required for success in integrated health delivery systems. Today many health care organizations are part of larger organizational entities, even if not fully integrated delivery networks. Thus, Longest's work is highly relevant for today's clinical leaders. His list of competencies includes conceptual, technical management/clinical, interpersonal/collaboration, political, commercial, and governance.

Longest's conceptual competency is closely related to prior definitions of the same name. In the area of technical management/clinical, Longest specifically mentions how important it is for senior health care managers to have knowledge of the clinical work done in their organizations. Similar expectations exist for clinical leaders in their areas of responsibility. Partnering and interorganizational relationships are new competencies mentioned in the interpersonal/collaboration category.

The last three competence categories are new additions, and although discussed in the context of senior leaders, bear important implications for all clinical leaders. Political competence relates to the impact that public and other health care policy decisions have on organizations and subunits. It is not unusual for clinical leaders to be active in the political arena for both their organizations and their professional societies or groups. Commercial competence includes both purchases and providers of care thinking about quality and cost of services; in fact, value may be defined as quality divided by price (Zelman, 1996). Increasingly, more attention is being paid to an episode of care across the care continuum rather that a judgment that in one setting or another (for example, acute care hospital vs. home care). The totality of outcomes and resource utilization is the new metric. Last, the governance competence speaks to establishing a clear organizational vision, fostering a culture to support that vision, and allocating the resources to achieve the vision in order to be accountable to the organization's stakeholders.

Additionally, the American Organization of Nurse Executives (AONE), published recommended leadership competencies (2005), that include communication/relationship management, knowledge of the healthcare environment, business skills/principles, and professionalism.

Research on Health Care Leadership Competencies

The findings of three studies of health care leaders provide an additional dimension to defining contemporary leadership competencies. Table 7.4 summarizes the studies. A two-part study by Ridenour (1996) sought to determine competencies essential for effective leadership by nurse executives in the year 2000. The eight competencies identified were developed into a tool for measuring nurse administrator competency. The eight domains of competence are quality improvement, shared visions, global approach, serving community, mastering change, team learning, managing customer relationships, and managing a diverse workforce. Scores on this tool were used to identify expertise and targeted priorities for training in a select group of clinical leaders.

A study by Byers (2001) investigated health care leadership, challenges, and future vision. As part of this study to identify critical leadership skills, senior nurses were surveyed in Florida health care organizations. With a total of 269 surveys returned, the most critical knowledge or skills for health care leaders were identified in order of importance as effective communication and interpersonal skills, government regulations/reimbursement, flexibility/ creativity, relationship building, change management, ability to vision and motivate, financial savvy, quality management, strategic planning and thinking, and political savvy.

One of the largest recent studies by VHA, Inc. (Gelinas et al., 1999) reported on the final segment of a national, three-part longitudinal study of the impact of organizational redesign on nurse executive leadership. The report addressed critical skills of health care nurse leaders in expanded roles from 444 nurse executives. The results of this study are particularly important because of the size of the study and national perspective. The findings covered 7 major areas.

Table 7.4   Leadership Competencies in Contemporary Research

Ridenour (1996)	Byers (2001)	VHA, Inc. (2000)
Quality improvement, shared visions, global approach, serving community, mastering change, team learning, managing customer relationships, and managing a diverse workforce	Effective communication and interpersonal skills, government regulations/ reimbursement, flexibility/ creativity, relationship building, change management, ability to vision and motivate, financial savvy, quality management, strategic planning and thinking, and political savvy	Customer needs and expectations, human resource management, care management systems, financial outcomes, data management, strategic visioning and planning, marketing initiatives, and continuous improvement skills

The first four findings reflect restructuring and refocusing of health care entities. Specifically, community hospital systems continue to redesign their systems, suggesting that organizational changes (including mergers, acquisitions, divorces, and restructuring) have become an ongoing management tool. Restructuring across the continuum of care is changing the face of health care, with increases in linkages to various outpatient or community entities. Patient satisfaction, quality and clinical outcomes, reduction of costs, and physician satisfaction are re-emphasized as the major evaluation criteria for system redesign result. And, not surprisingly then, patient satisfaction has moved to the forefront as a major goal for nursing/patient care executives and joins reducing or controlling costs as top priority goals to be achieved.

The last three findings speak to internal changes to achieve and support those just presented. Integration of services and coordination across departments continues to be the most highly consistent feature of system redesign. Chief Nurse Officers report more than doubling the number of departments for which they are accountable, from 14 in 1993 to over 30 in 1998. And last, high priority learning needs (or important leadership competencies) for clinical services executives include implementing clinical improvement, understanding finance, using pathways and tools, change management expertise, understanding managed care, and advanced teambuilding skills.

The study concludes with a proposal to identify the competencies for nurse executives (and by extension clinical leaders) for the 21st century. The subsequently proposed leadership competencies (VHA, Inc., 2000) are customer needs and expectations, human resource management, care management systems, financial outcomes, data management, strategic visioning and planning, marketing initiatives, and continuous improvement skills.

COMPETENCIES FOR CLINICAL LEADERSHIP IN THE 21ST CENTURY

We propose seven essential competencies, largely drawn from the work by VHA, Inc. and the authors cited above, to position the clinical leader for success in the 21st century.

These competencies are congruent with the values and approaches of the three lenses presented earlier, transformational leadership, Leadership IQ, and complexity science. Table 7.5 summarizes each competency.

While some adaptation of the competency statements may be required depending upon the specific services of a given area or unit, these competencies are proposed as the core for clinical leaders. Each of these competencies is described briefly in the remainder of this chapter and then discussed in detail in subsequent chapters of this section.

Table 7.5   Multi-dimensional Leadership Model Role Competencies for Clinical Managers

1. **Customer Needs and Expectations**
   To collaborate in the design and delivery of care services that meet or exceed customer expectations.

2. **Visioning and Strategic Planning**
   To create and communicate a shared compelling vision of the future along with developing a strategic plan for action to achieve that vision for the clinical unit.

3. **Managing Care Across the Continuum**
   To foster systems to coordinate care across health care settings to promote optimal client outcomes and cost-effective, resource-efficient care.

4. **Improving Quality and Performance**
   To use information and quality tools to continuously improve performance and create a culture of quality.

5. **Human Resource Management**
   To manage a talented diverse workforce in an environment that fosters staff satisfaction, growth, and achievement of clinical unit goals.

6. **Marketing Initiatives**
   To develop innovative products and services that meet needs of existing and potential customers and participate in the promotion of those services.

7. **Financial Outcomes**
   To employ financial management principles and techniques to serve as an effective steward of resources in fulfilling the clinical unit mission.

Customer Needs and Expectations

When we use the term *customers*, we are usually referring to clients or patients and their families. For some clinical areas, however, major customers might also include physicians or others in the organization. In short, customers are those whom we exist to serve.

While it may be difficult to imagine now, only in the last 20 years or so have health care organizations seriously considered the true needs, expectations, and preferences of clients. Some would argue that we continue to struggle with this concept today. A hallmark in addressing customers is to eliminate the belief that health care leaders know what customers need and want without asking them. Measuring customer satisfaction has become a community standard as well as a regulatory expectation.

Measuring patient satisfaction has grown increasingly sophisticated, and numerous proprietary surveys are available that boast strong validity and reliability. Their use provides for extensive benchmarking of similar institutions. One of the most effective ways to enhance patient satisfaction is for senior leadership and clinical managers to emphasize the need to manage customer expectations. When clients have unrealistic views of what health care services can provide they are bound to be dissatisfied. Clarifying and negotiating what can be provided has been shown to be of value in improving patient satisfaction scores (Baker, 1998).

Health care providers are sometimes sensitive to how client satisfaction is measured. In their view clients can only report their satisfaction with the service aspects of care and some of the clinical outcomes, because professional knowledge is required to assess the quality of care. The increasing availability and use of evidence-based guidelines and outcomes may help to resolve this concern.

Almost all agree that the design, implementation, and continuous improvement of health care delivery models and services must be based on valid assessments. These assessments should address expectations, and preferences to better serve customers and to assure that health care organizations achieve their service and financial goals.

Visioning and Strategic Planning

The most important foundation of a health-care organization's success is visionary leadership, for the whole organization, and for each unit or departmental area. A vision is an image of a possible and desirable future state for the organization or unit. It must be realistic, attainable, credible, challenging, and attractive to those in the organization. Most important, the vision should be known and internalized by everyone in the organization and serve as a guiding light to illuminate the desired pathway.

To create a vision that meets these criteria requires sound analysis of the internal and external environments as well as understanding the historical (hindsight) and evolving (foresight) conditions. Both external and internal factors significantly affect the ability of the organization to achieve its vision.

The ability of the clinical leader to embrace the overall organizational vision and translate that into a coherent, clear unit vision is essential. A vision should guide decision making, resource allocation, and change objectives to ensure that each of these promotes progress toward the stated vision (often referred to as alignment) across the organization or unit. The unit vision should address client care management systems and outcomes and the role of staff in providing client services in a satisfying and meaningful environment.

Strategic planning or thinking is the systematic process used in most organizations to develop specific goals and action plans that will move the organization toward realization of its vision. In health care settings clinical leaders may have input into the overall strategic plan. They can also use the strategic planning process at the unit level.

There are numerous approaches to strategic planning; most include assessments of the internal and external environments, a SWOT analysis (strengths, weaknesses, opportunities, threats), development of strategic initiatives, implementation plans for the strategic initiatives, and periodic evaluation of the results to check progress and verify final outcomes.

Managing Care Across the Continuum

Few would identify the United States health care system as a model for health promotion and coordination of services. In fact, many providers and patients say that we have an illness- or disease-based system. Most resources are still consumed by acute care hospital settings, but it is important to consider the totality of care for a given condition of problem. Also referred to as an episode of care, this would involve consideration of the outcomes and costs of care for all care services. For example, if a joint replacement is performed on a 72-year-old man, he would likely have pre-surgical testing, an acute care hospital stay of 3–5 days, perhaps a week of care at a rehabilitation hospital, and then home nursing and physical therapy for a period of weeks. In this type of case, assessing costs and outcomes for only the hospital stay or the rehabilitation period would not provide a good picture of all of the resources required for treatment of this diagnosis.

Whether functioning in a truly integrated health care delivery system or with various loosely linked network agreements, the clinical leader must consider what happens to clients before and after their service or care encounter in your area or setting. On the quality side of the equation, there is strong documentation of the positive impact of health maintenance, screening, and promotion activities on the development and/or severity of various diagnoses. Similarly, appropriate follow-up care at home or as appropriate in an extended care facility can decrease length of stays in hospitals and deliver better clinical outcomes with fewer complications (such as infection).

Consider the impact of improper preparation for an outpatient diagnostic test. If the test cannot be performed properly, the client and provider are dissatisfied, revenue and productivity are diminished unexpectedly, therapeutic interventions may be delayed or compromised, and the overall cost of care for this episode increases.

From the client perspective, lack of coordination and knowledge of patient needs and conditions compromises, and in many cases, endangers people. Patient and family frustrations with a fragmented and seemingly uncaring system are commonly reported. So both providers and patients are seeking seamless interfaces among health-care providers, settings, and services.

Achieving these seamless interfaces among providers and settings requires a clear definition of the continuum of services available for a given patient population in a specific region, defined models for coordinating and evaluating care, and the use of evidence-based best practices to deliver high-quality and cost-effective services. Specifically, the contributions of case management and disease management have been prominent in recent literature because these activities include coordination and communication about care needs and decision making. Again, the importance of current and accurate assessments of provider performance and client needs and outcomes (clinical, functional, satisfaction, and costs at a minimum) should be reemphasized as we try to improve care. This information may also lead to evaluation and improvement of reimbursement structures that benefit both payers and clients.

Clinical managers will need to develop and implement models for managing care including identifying roles and responsibilities. Information technology and access to relevant data about evidence-based clinical care protocols will be needed to assure high-quality, cost-effective services.

Improving Quality and Performance

Today's health care environment requires constant attention to improving quality and performance measures to meet societal health care needs and at the same time remaining competitive and successful. The clinical leader is the translator of organizational approaches to quality improvement (QI) and plays a major role in identifying priorities for improvement, establishing and maintaining quality standards, and ensuring the safety, efficacy, and effectiveness of care.

The quality movement has matured in health care organizations with a goal of creating cultures of quality that focus on outcomes and continuous improvement. The tools and techniques of QI that rely heavily on teams and data to drive improvement decisions have demonstrated their potential in health care settings. Additionally, regulatory and accrediting agencies have launched aggressive initiatives to measure and publicly report comparative quality and outcome information.

Clinical process improvement and evidence-based care practices are critical skill sets for health care leaders; they enhance QI efforts through multidisciplinary teamwork that relies on data or evidence for creating best practices.

Clinical leaders and their staffs are at the heart of these efforts where the care is actually delivered. Commitment to continuous improvement in the clinical and administrative domains not only increases quality and efficiency but can reenergize and increase satisfaction for staff and clients.

Human Resource Management

Most of the work of clinical leaders involves working with other people to achieve unit and organizational goals. Managing human resources is a complex skill set that is facilitated by a systematic approach. We present a model for organizing your activities relating to human resource management to help you. The model includes work analysis, staffing, recruitment and selection of staff, staff development, performance evaluation, staff retention, and rewards. Information about disciplinary actions and terminations is also included.

One of the most important goals is for clinical leaders to work collaboratively with staff to create a unit vision for a positive and productive work environment that is satisfying to staff and embraces continuous quality improvement goals. Strategies for developing and achieving a vision for the unit are provided for your use.

Marketing Initiatives

Marketing is a critical competency for clinical leaders in an increasingly competitive health care arena. Marketing takes into account customer needs and preferences as you create innovative products and services and how you promote them.

Clinical leaders have unique and valuable perspectives on current operations and care delivery. When matched with information about existing and potential customer needs and preferences, clinical leaders along with their staffs and other key disciplines can use QI methods to design new approaches to service delivery.

Marketing essentials related to the consumer, the product, and the message are explored in the context of health care services with a focus on innovation, access, and quality.

Financial Outcomes

The role of clinical leaders in achieving desired financial outcomes continues to grow in importance due to ongoing concerns regarding escalating costs of health care. The use of financial management tools, techniques, and strategies to control costs and to enhance the value of services at the unit level is essential. Familiarity with the financial position of your organization and related financial goals provides the context for your decision making at the unit level.

Also important are knowing who the major purchasers or payers of your services are and how revenue is generated both through your area, if applicable, and throughout your organization. As managed care practices have permeated the health care industry, clinical leaders need to increase their knowledge and confidence regarding contract requirements and procedures. An enhanced perspective on financial matters should position you to be an effective steward of your resources to fulfill the clinical unit and organizational missions.

In summary, these seven leadership competencies comprise the core skills needed by transformational clinical leaders for the 21st century. As you build your skill levels within each, you can expect to see positive outcomes and improved performance. Depending on your role and responsibilities, other leadership competencies may also be critical for your success. If so, add them to this list as you design and implement your professional development plan.

Although not included as a specific competency, we would emphasize the importance of maintaining a healthy work/life balance. Your ability to create this balance will preserve and renew your energy, enrich your life, and provide a positive model for your staff and colleagues. Refer back to Chapter 6 ("Managing Personal Resources") on a regular basis if this topic is a challenge for you.

APPLICATION EXERCISES

Specific applications and case scenarios are presented at the end of the following chapters on the seven leadership competencies. Here we focus on the competencies as a whole.

1. Using the seven competencies for clinical leadership in the 21st century, write a sentence next to each that describes an important activity that you are or would be responsible for within your current or desired role.

2. Which two or three competencies are most important in your current or projected next position and why?

3. Are there any major activities or responsibilities related to your role as leader that cannot be reasonably categorized within the seven competencies? If yes, consider why that is and what other competencies are needed for success.

REFERENCES

American Organization of Nurse Executives. (2005). AONE nurse executive competencies, *Nurse Leader*, February, 50–56.

Baker, S. K. (1998). *Managing expectations: The art of finding and keeping loyal patients*. San Francisco: Jossey-Bass.

Bennis, W., & Nanus, B. (1985, 1997). *Leaders: The strategies for taking charge*. New York: Harper & Row.

Byers, J. F. (2001). Voices from the field: Health care leadership, challenges, and future vision. Research abstract, T. L. Carroll, ed. In *Nursing Administrative Quarterly*, *25* (4), 87–90.

Contino, D. S. (2004). Leadership competencies: Knowledge, skills, and aptitudes nurses need to lead organizations effectively. *Critical Care Nurse*, *24* (3), 52–64.

Gelinas, L. S., Sullivan, D. T., Newton, G., Manthey, M., & Seidel, B. (1999). *The impact of organizational redesign on nurse executive leadership, Part III*. Irving, TX: VHA, Inc.

Katz, R. L. (1974). Skills of an effective administrator. *Harvard Business Review, 52* (5), 90–102.

Katz, R. L., & Kahn, D. (1978). *The social psychology of organizations (2nd ed.)*. New York: John Wiley & Sons.

Longest, B. B. (1998). Managerial competence at senior levels of integrated delivery systems. *Journal of Healthcare Management, 43* (2), 115–132.

Mintzberg, H. (1973). *The nature of managerial work*. New York: Harper & Row.

Mintzberg, H. (1990). The manager's job: Folklore and fact. *Harvard Business Review, 68* (2), March–April.

Perra, B. M. (2001). Leadership: The key to quality outcomes. *Journal of Nursing Care Quality, 15* (2), 68–73.

Ridenour, J. E. (1996). Measuring competencies: Development of the administrator competency survey. *Seminars for Nurse Managers, 4* (2), 98–106.

Schein, E. (1975). How "career anchors" hold executives to their career paths. *Personnel, 52* (3), 11–24.

Simon, H. (1976). *Administrative behavior (3rd ed.)*. New York: The Free Press.

Tomey, A. H. (2004). *Guide to nursing management and leadership*. St. Louis: Mosby, p. 169.

VHA, Inc. (2000, April). *Revolutionizing the future of nursing care: Defining the role of the chief nursing officer in the 21st century*. A white paper developed by the VHA National Nursing Leadership Council.

Zaleznik, A. (1977). Managers and leaders: Are they different? *Harvard Business Review, 55* (3), 67–68.

Zelman, W. A. (1996). *The changing healthcare marketplace: Private ventures, public interests*. San Francisco: Jossey-Bass.

CHAPTER 8

Customer Needs and Expectations

Michael J. Emery

*To collaborate in the design and delivery of care services
that meet or exceed customer expectations.*

───── **CHAPTER QUESTIONS** ─────

1. Who are the various "consumer groups" in health care and how do their motives differ?
2. How is consumerism different in the health care context?
3. What are the best ways to determine consumer satisfaction in health care?
4. What are the most important elements of consumer satisfaction in health care?
5. What are our legal and ethical obligations relative to our patients or their families as "consumers"?

INTRODUCTION

The culture and economy of the United States have combined to create an era of consumerism that is not previously paralleled. Focus on the consumer and attention to consumer satisfaction has risen as consumers:

- Have demonstrated that they have the resources necessary to purchase
- Have demanded choice in what they purchase
- Can assess the value (cost compared to quality) of what they purchase, and
- Have demonstrated willingness to take their business elsewhere when they are not satisfied

As a result, consumerism has flourished. Marketing efforts seek to attract increasingly sophisticated buyers who have choice and are willing to use it.

Consumers have become more willing to bring the market-place principles of purchasing power, choice, and selection based on value from traditional marketplace settings to public service settings such as public education, social

113

welfare, and health care. In this chapter we explore the role and impact of consumer orientation in health and determine how, as a clinical manager, you work to address the consumer needs and the expectations that have become part of today's health care environment.

CONSUMERISM IN HEALTH CARE

Who is the consumer in health care? Clearly this includes the patient and the patient's family as the direct recipients of health care services, but consumerism in health care is more complex than that. When we consider Who is the purchaser? we should also consider the employer, the insurance company, and even the government. All are in some way involved in the consumption of health care services because they receive or pay for these services. In this chapter, however, the discussion focuses on the primary consumers (patients and their families).

Factors Contributing to Consumerism

Consumerism in health care has been promoted by the same forces found in other sectors of our society. Health care consumers expect higher levels of service, have greater access to health care information, and seek to play a greater role in their health care decisions (Mallory, 2003; Scandlen, 2004). Beyond this, our society continues to debate the question of whether or not health care is a public service or a business, and has done so long after other nations have declared health care to be a public service (Jones, 2000).

Two additional factors in health care in the United States have further encouraged this consumer orientation: managed care and the patient-centered approach to care. Managed care, implemented in the late 1980s and evolving to the present day, is a system of health care management that seeks to control health care costs and sustain quality by sharing risk between providers and consumers of care. Thus, consumers are encouraged to be more committed participants in the decisions, and outcomes of health care (McLoughlin & Leatherman, 2003). Consumers have become motivated to be more informed about health care choices and to participate more actively in the decision-making process. While managed care was implemented for the purpose of controlling health care costs, one of the significant side effects of these past 25 years of managed care has been to produce more knowledgeable, assertive, and wary consumers of health care services.

The patient-centered approach to health care was first developed as a pediatric patient-care model for children with chronic disabilities in the 1970s.

Consumers (children, their parents, and other providers) demanded more openness in the decision-making process and a role in that decision making. Patient-centered care conceptualizes the patient at the center and the various other services and providers surrounding the patient in a way that keeps all focused on the centrality of identified patient needs. This included priorities for various health care services and a focus on patient outcomes as factors that weighed most heavily on clinical decision making (Berry et al., 2003). As a result, patients were allowed and encouraged to advocate for their priorities in terms of services they received and outcomes they expected. In the case of minor children, parents and teachers served as the child's advocate in making these demands. While patient-centered care was an approach intended to improve the quality of care and patient/advocate satisfaction, a side effect of this approach was to reinforce the consumer orientation that we are familiar with in other sectors of our society.

The Growing Trend of Consumerism

In the past two decades, consumer orientation in health care has increased as the health care industry has become more business oriented rather than service oriented. The demands of consumers have become particularly apparent in issues of consumer choice, access to services, quality of care, and affordability of care (Coddington et al., 2001). Insurance companies have made numerous adjustments in their policies to satisfy consumers and to compete more successfully with those purchasing health insurance, typically employers. Beyond this, health care consumers have demonstrated an increasing interest in the characteristics of their health care providers and the corporations in which they work. Kizer (2001) reports that beyond the elements of patient care quality mentioned above, consumers are also concerned about measures of clinical performance and public accountability. Consumers are seeking information on their own about the effectiveness of treatments, the performance of their health care providers, and the rankings of health care institutions and companies.

Consumers have developed a significant appreciation for the information that is increasingly available on all aspects of health and health care through the Internet and other sources. Patients increasingly understand that health care is a risky business, and that one way in which they can improve their chances for a favorable outcome is to become informed and to participate more actively in their own health care decisions. This understandable skepticism about health care combined with ready access to health information has rapidly expanded the knowledge of many patients in today's health care system, and is likely to provide an even more informed and demanding consumer population in the future (Walsh, 2003).

Responding to Consumerism

Many institutions have responded by reconsidering the role of the consumer in health care. Institutional mission statements have been revised to reflect the importance of patient satisfaction and consumer orientation in the operations of the institution. The patient's bill of rights has become a standard fixture in hospitals, nursing homes, and rehabilitation centers where patients and their families, often disconcerted by events leading to hospitalization or otherwise reluctant in these settings, are reminded of what they can expect from the institution and how to express their dissatisfaction if they feel that these rights are not provided. Even in the more competitive private sector of health care, clinics and offices often share the comments of satisfied patients and offer commitments to patients about the satisfaction that would-be patients can expect.

Finally, patient care services always have the potential to lead to unsuccessful outcomes, failed procedures, or unsatisfied patients. Some in health care have adopted the approach of other prudent businesses, where strategies to provide quick and effective remedies are a part of the plan for service. Communication is the key to this process. It needs to be timely, honest, and demonstrate concern. In measures of patient satisfaction, patients are more likely to be satisfied if they feel as though they were kept informed and if they received the care that was necessary. Mistakes are inevitable in some cases some of the time. How errors are dealt with, not whether or not they happen, determine how the providers will be judged by patients and others.

As a clinical manager, you are ideally positioned to monitor the experience and the outcomes as seen by the customer and you have the authority to address shortcomings or errors in patient service. The concept of service recovery is to continually assess the delivery of service and to correct or resolve errors or shortcomings in the delivery of service. The task of service recovery is essential in health care services, as errors and omissions are not entirely avoidable. The clinical manager can be highly effective in service recovery, as they can observe, assess, and intervene as may be necessary.

ASSESSING CONSUMER NEEDS

While this chapter focuses on assessing consumer needs, such an assessment is part of a larger assessment of patient outcomes. The consumer is in the best position to assess some aspects of patient care, but not all aspects. Patient satisfaction, therefore, has become one measure of patient outcomes but not the only one. Outcomes of patient care also include a comparison to practice standards and expected outcome standards (clinical effectiveness), and the resources used to achieve these outcomes (resource management) (Campbell et al., 2000). All contribute to a comprehensive outcome assessment.

Patient Satisfaction

Patient satisfaction, while only a part of the patient outcome, is important for several reasons. Patients who are satisfied with their care are:

- More likely to continue to use that institution for their continuing care
- More compliant with treatment programs
- Have fewer malpractice claims, and are
- More likely to promote the facility to other patients (Shelton, 2000).

It is therefore important that each health professional promote the perspective of the patient and include the patient's perspective in the clinical decision-making process (Hughes, 2003).

Two approaches to identifying the patients' assessment of their care have been used successfully: patient satisfaction surveys and patient complaints (See Table 8.1). Patient satisfaction measurement instruments are typically designed to address a specific practice setting, and the tools used vary widely (Woodring et al., 2003; Fielden et al., 2003; Aspinal et al., 2003; Jennings & Loan, 1999). This creates difficulty in comparing across settings and institutions but does allow institutions to compare themselves using the same tool over time. Patient satisfaction depends on many factors but most often includes access to care, communication with health care providers, effectiveness of interventions, and efficiency of treatment. The role of other factors and their influence on patient satisfaction is not fully understood and the subject of various theoretical models of patient satisfaction (Hudak et al., 2004; Williams, 2002).

One way to address the difficulty in comparing separate customized patient satisfaction tools is to consider standardized patient satisfaction instruments. A variety of tools have become available in recent years, as patient surveys have become more popular and their role in systematically assessing clinical satisfaction and perceptions of care has been recognized. There are numerous proprietary patient satisfaction surveys now available from consulting firms and other business services in health care. Two of these have captured a major portion of the market: those from Press Ganey and the Picker Institute. Both have extensive reliability and validity data supporting their use. Press Ganey incorporates many of the so-called hotel or guest services in their assessment. Picker Institute surveys take a somewhat different approach, focusing more on the care and caring. Both have assisted many health care organizations in making improvements and designing new services based on client feedback and benchmarking.

Table 8.1   Measuring Patient Satisfaction

Type	Description	Purpose
Patient Satisfaction Survey	• Written or computerized • Open or closed-ended questions • Can be completed independently	• Access to care • Communication with health care providers • Effectiveness of interventions • Efficiency of treatment
Patient Complaints	• Verbal or written • Formative or summative • Patients/family/others	• Achievement of minimum standards • Problematic aspects of service delivery
Focus Groups	• Small consumer groups • In-depth questioning or discussion	• Identifies consumer recommendations and strategies • Time-consuming but yields rich information
Needs Assessment	• Survey or interviews • Can be applied to groups or individuals • Designed to elicit patient needs or demands	• Prioritizes consumer needs • Links patient needs to quality of life issues
"Walking Around"	• Being physically present to patients and staff • Asking questions and listening • Observing operations for positive and negative aspects	• Informal, less threatening communication with consumers • Provides useful insights/interpretation • Demonstrates the emotional significance of the consumer concern or complaint

Patient Complaints

The use of patient complaints as a measure of patient satisfaction is an indirect measure. While it identifies what patients may be upset about, it does not necessarily mean that correcting these issues increases satisfaction. For example, a patient may complain about a hospital bill, but better communication and more timely care may be what would make the patient more satisfied, not a reduction in the hospital bill. For this reason, monitoring of patient complaints may be more useful when measuring achievement of a minimal acceptable standard or identifying the most troubling components of a delivery system (Born & Query, 2004).

Focus Groups

The use of patient focus groups is another effective tool in assessing consumer needs. This approach includes the use of semistructured, guiding questions with a small (6–12 persons) group of consumers. Focus groups allow for the opportunity for follow-up questions, determining group consensus or not, and exploring what solution may be most acceptable to the consumer group. The process is more time consuming and labor intensive for both the institution and the consumer. Careful selection of a focus group is important as the goal is to achieve a representative sample of consumers. This method is useful when assessing a new service, understanding in greater detail the issues of patient dissatisfaction, and other situations in which richer, detailed information regarding patient satisfaction is needed.

Needs Assessment

Needs assessment is a planning tool that has historically been used to plan for the needs of a population of people. More recently this tool has been used on an individual patient basis (Wright et al., 1998). Needs assessments for a population typically were used to measure prevalence of various patient illnesses, risk factors, and patient complaints, which were then interpreted by practitioners and others into a statement of need. Increasingly, needs assessments are now focused on the needs as identified by the patient or consumer groups. This allows the consumer group to determine the relative importance of competing needs and to guide the priorities for addressing these needs. This sorting of needs provides for a more comprehensive measure of quality of life. Patients can express what, in their view, is the most troubling aspect of an illness, the greatest problem that they face, or the most disturbing of the many symptoms that they may experience. Quality of life as reflected in these needs assessments is typically influenced by physical functioning, psychological processes, social and economical concerns, as well as patient beliefs and spirituality (Davidson et al., 2004).

Needs assessment can be used for both individual patients and whole communities, but is most useful when it includes an assessment by the consumer of how the various elements of his health status interact to create a hierarchy of health needs. Interventions then are most likely to have meaningful impact on the patient's quality of life.

As a clinical manager, you should consider each of these tools to assess patient satisfaction as you construct a process to provide feedback from the patient to you, your staff, and the leaders of the institution.

Assessment by "Walking Around"

While each of these methods of assessing patient needs and satisfaction provides useful information to assess a provider's or an institution's performance, each is engineered in some ways and therefore somewhat contrived. In balance, another important tool to assess patient/family needs is to simply be available and attentive to them—clinical management by "walking around."

Consumers are usually more than willing to talk about what they like and don't like, what worked and what did not, and what they are most concerned about. What they need is a listener who is genuinely interested and who reinforces the notion that their assessment of their needs and expectations is valued. Reinforcing the role that patients should play in the assessment of patient outcomes is not always easy in a delivery system that moves at a rapid pace and is rife with more quantitative and scientific data upon which to base patient decisions. The centrality of the patient in patient care, however, would argue that we must take the time to listen to a patient and to affirm the significance of his perspective in determining needs, establishing treatment priorities, and assessing the effectiveness of the interventions. In the end, decisions that include the patient's perspective are most likely to influence quality of life (Williams, 2002).

MANAGING CONSUMER NEEDS AND EXPECTATIONS

The Patient Bill of Rights

In most health care institutions today the patient's bill of rights is prominently displayed for all to view. It identifies what patients can expect in their interaction with health care providers, and it clarifies how they can best assert these rights in the patient care delivery process. Indirectly, the patient's bill of rights provides for a standard of patient expectations. Patients and providers know what is fair to expect and what is not. For the clinical manager, this becomes an important reference point, and should be referred to often with patients and staff. The institution may also have, through its mission statement, a performance standard that provides a reference point for patient expectations (e.g., Patients can expect to have their questions answered in a timely way). Without such performance standards, expectations and therefore patient satisfaction can vary widely among patients and families. Equally important, these standards become tools to ensure fairness across patients and families, as the provider and the institution seek to meet their responsibility to all patients, not just a few.

Achieving Patient Satisfaction

As stated earlier, patient satisfaction is multifaceted and varies from patient to patient. The most significant elements of patient satisfaction include access to care, communication with health care providers, effectiveness of interventions, and efficiency of treatment. Patient examination and treatment activities that can be explained in this context are much more likely to be accepted by patients. As a clinical manager, you must ensure that:

- The daily routine and services provided by your staff are linked to these patient expectations
- Patients and families understand this linkage, and
- Staff members take the time to listen to the patient's assessment of his own need.

This will guide the priorities of treatment intervention.

Care that improves the quality of life is, by a patient's definition, quality care. Such quality of care will determine patient satisfaction. So, to borrow from a popular advertising slogan, "Patient satisfaction is Job One!"

As mentioned earlier, meeting patient expectations leads to patient satisfaction. To ensure that patient and family expectations are reasonable and equitable, we have tools such as the patient's bill of rights and institutional mission statements. Patients must be aware of these if reasonable patient expectations are to be anticipated. Health care providers are well served by taking the time to be sure that patients are aware of and understand these statements of rights and expectations. This will allow patients to both identify when reasonable expectations are not met, but also when they are exceeded. As a clinical manager, you need to be attentive not only to those instances when the institution falls short of patient expectations, but also when it exceeds patient expectations. Patient satisfaction can also be significantly influenced by the patients being aware that their expectations have been exceeded by a provider, a service, or an institution.

Solving Patient Problems

Patient satisfaction is not synonymous with the absence of problems. Indeed, problems are the very reasons that one seeks health care and so health care, by definition, is a problem-oriented enterprise. Satisfaction is determined by how problems are identified and resolved and by whom. So, managing patient satisfaction is a process of identifying, assessing, and fixing patient problems. For the patient, these are not just health problems, but also include social, economic, spiritual, and health system problems. Health care workers at all levels must be prepared to

- triage such problems,
- recognize what is within and beyond their individual scope of competence and responsibility,
- identify who can address the problem, and
- initiate a referral for the problem to the appropriate person in a timely fashion.

In this way, consumer or patient satisfaction becomes everyone's responsibility. Satisfaction is determined not by the absence of problems but by the way the institution and its staff identified, assessed, and resolved the problem.

ROLE OF THE MANAGER IN MEETING CONSUMER NEEDS AND EXPECTATIONS

As stated, managing the consumers' needs and expectations is everyone's responsibility in a health care institution. One could argue, however, that this management role falls particularly to the leaders of the various patient care teams, clinical units, and service areas (i.e., health care microsystems). Beyond this, the clinical manager has several unique responsibilities to ensure that consumer needs are met (see Table 8.2).

Know the Patient's Perspective

First, the clinical manager is best positioned to serve as the patient's voice when the patient is not present. Many clinical decisions are made in the absence of patients; yet their perspective is essential. As a clinical manager, through your own communication and observation, as well as that of your staff, you are ideally positioned to raise the concerns, questions, and priorities that the patient has expressed and to ensure that these receive appropriate consideration in the clinical decision-making process. This clinical management characteristic is called empathy. Not to be confused with sympathy, *empathy* is the ability to assume the perspective, the point of view, of another person and to understand and value that perspective despite your own knowledge or beliefs. Empathy means to understand and assume the values, priorities, and the positions of another person for the purpose of representing his perspective in the best possible way. The clinical manager is uniquely positioned to assume this empathetic role. Empathy also should not be confused with paternalism, which means making judgments on behalf of another person based on your knowledge or skills. Generally, health care providers exercise a great deal of paternalism on their patients' behalf in an effort to be helpful. We

Table 8.2   Clinical Manager's Role in Assessing Consumer Needs

Know the patient's perspective	• Identify concerns, questions, and priorities of the patient • Understand patient values and beliefs (empathy) • Avoid paternalism
Serve as the patient's voice	• Speak on the patient's behalf • Assure that the patient's perspective is considered in decision making
Ensure adherence to policies and procedures	• Recognize and enforce applicable policies and procedures • Consider applicable laws • Understand moral/ethic elements of decision making • Ensure adherence to these guidelines
Promote ethical discernment	• Involve experts as may be required in the clinical decision-making process • Promote sufficient use of time in arriving at clinical decisions • Ensure participation of patient and family as is appropriate

should recognize, however, that this paternalism takes authority and control away from patients and gives it to the provider. Empathy rather than paternalism should be our goal when speaking on a patient's behalf.

Serve as the Patient's Voice

Second, the clinical manager serves as the patient's voice. Once the patient's values, concerns, and priorities are known, the clinical manager must give voice to these. Patients may not always be present, able, or confident enough to voice their perspective. As a clinical manager, you can assure that their voice is heard and receives the appropriate weight in the process of making clinical decisions. It is important also that patients know that their perspective is being voiced by another person on their behalf.

Ensure Adherence to Policies/Procedures

Third, the clinical manager, as the leader closest to the patient, must assure that policies and procedures, laws, and ethical principles are adhered to in the process of patient care decision making. As a clinical manager, you are always accountable at some level to authorities for adherence to these various expectations. The clinical manager is most likely to be in a position to recognize and correct situations that threaten to violate these expectations. Perhaps most important, as a clinical manager, you have the authority to stop, redirect, or revise action plans that may violate these various expectations.

Promote Ethical Discernment

Finally, promoting ethical discernment in patient care decisions is the responsibility of and requires the support of the clinical manager. Health care decision making is full of ethical conflict and dilemmas in today's delivery system. Institutions have increased their resources in this area by adding ethicists in residence, ethics teams, and staff training to help promote careful, thoughtful deliberation when faced with two competing harms or goods for the patient. As a clinical manager, you can recognize the need to bring the necessary resources into play in discerning the best course of action for such patients. The clinical manager need not be the ethics expert but must be able to identify such challenges, bring the necessary people and resources together, and ensure that actions are not taken without careful deliberation.

Each of these clinical manager responsibilities contributes to meeting patient's expectations and promoting patient satisfaction. As a clinical manager, you have the opportunity and the authority to promote these within the clinical decision-making process, with the goal of greater patient satisfaction and quality of life, as well as providing a distinctive role model for your staff in patient representation and inclusion in the clinical decision-making process.

SCENARIO

Marie is a clinical manager in an acute care hospital in a small city. Her hospital has just merged with a competitor across town. Marie has been asked to lead a cardiac rehabilitation program that was inherited from the competing institution. The cardiac rehabilitation program has operated in a substandard fashion for several years. This is widely known by providers and patients alike, based on patient complaints, generally poor patient compliance, staff turnover, and questionable patient outcomes. Marie has been asked to lead the "re-invention" of this service to serve the newly merged parent organization and the patients of both hospitals. Expectations of her performance include (1) better patient satisfaction measures, (2) demonstrated clinical effectiveness of the service, and (3) reasonable resource constraints in the transformation of this service. Reassessment of this program will occur in one year. The current staff is frustrated and rather demoralized by past program performance, yet they are optimistic about the new program leadership and the changes that Marie will lead in the program.

In Marie's strategy to address patient needs and expectations, she decides to form a focus group of previous patients who have used the service and a separate focus group of current staff for the service. Her goal is to prioritize the concerns or problems that these groups experienced and identify strategies for the new service that will minimize or avoid these concerns. Ultimately, this information will contribute to a new vision statement for the clinical unit.

In addition, she has reviewed patient satisfaction instruments from similar types of clinical services and has recommended adopting a patient satisfaction instrument that will focus on patient access, communication with providers, effectiveness of interventions, and efficiency of the service. Finally, during the startup of the new service, Marie has decided to organize her schedule so that she can spend some time just being in the patient treatment area so that she can talk informally with patients and their families to assess how the new service is being received and hear suggestions from these patients and their families.

With the newly constituted treatment team (herself and existing staff), Marie plans to meet frequently at the beginning of the planning phase of the new service to develop program goals, methods to measure the achievement of these goals, and activities that will include patient feedback of program goal achievement and efficiency of the operation.

SCENARIO ANALYSIS

Two important transformational leadership principles are relevant to this situation. First, Marie has stated the need for a vision for the unit. This vision must be shared among the unit staff and achievable. It must move the new cardiac rehab program toward the goals that the institution has indicated: (1) better patient satisfaction measures, (2) demonstrated clinical effectiveness of the service, and (3) reasonable resource constraints in the transformation of this service. Marie has developed two focus groups to help shape this vision statement and to guide the program toward a higher level of quality. The second transformational leadership principle important here is the need for self-esteem of the current staff. Marie has engaged the staff in the development of a new vision for the cardiac rehab service, and is seeking to invest the staff in achieving the institutional goals for the new program by being actively involved in its transformation. Meeting these goals will help staff self-esteem and increase their pride in being part of an effective clinical service. A vision for the reinvented service and enhancement of staff self-esteem will be important ingredients for the success of this service.

Two guiding principles for Leadership IQ are particularly important in this scenario. First, Marie has the benefit of being seen as an achiever by the institution that selected her and by the clinical staff who are looking to her for positive change. This confidence and opportunity gives Marie important momentum to move the clinical service in a positive direction. People are trusting that she will achieve change, and that confidence is half the battle. Marie is seizing that opportunity to initiate change in a swift and participatory way. Second, Marie has recognized the importance of being customer oriented by including past patients in her focus group, asking them what was good and what needs to be corrected. Ultimate success in this unit depends on customer satisfaction, and Marie has engaged these consumers in the reinvention process for the clinical service.

Complexity science suggests that relationships and connectedness are an important component of any health care system. Marie has chosen to be actively "out and about" in the new service area to make connections between herself and her new staff, and to connect consumers to this change process as well. The previous lack of success of the service is related to several interacting factors: poor staff morale, patient dissatisfaction, and inadequate treatment outcomes. The interaction of these problems requires Marie to engage all the significant players in this environment. Even more important is Marie's recognition that these clinical service problems are interactive, so to affect one of the problem areas she must affect all of them.

APPLICATION EXERCISES

1. In your own clinical unit, identify the sources of information regarding consumer satisfaction. Do the tools that your institution uses answer your most important customer satisfaction questions? Should you consider one of the proprietary patient satisfaction tools for your unit?

2. How does your clinical unit or institution monitor patient complaints? Are these assessed in some systematic way? Consider designing a system to review, assess, and respond to patient complaints.

3. Review any recent needs assessments that your institution has conducted. Do these include a patient perspective? If so, what are the priority needs as expressed by these patient data?

REFERENCES

Aspinal, F., Addington-Hall, J., Hughes, R., & Higginson, I. J. (2003). Using satisfaction to measure the quality of palliative care: A review of the literature. *Journal of Advanced Nursing, 42* (4), 324–339.

Berry, L. L., Seiders, K., & Wilder, S. S. (2003). Innovations in access to care: A patient-centered approach. *Annals of Internal Medicine, 139* (7), 568–574.

Born, P. H., & Query, J. T. (2004). Health maintenance organization (HMO) performance and consumer complaints: An empirical study of frustrating HMO activities. *Hospital Topics: Research and Perspectives on Healthcare, 82* (1), 2–9.

Campbell, S. M., Roland, M. O., & Buetow, S. A. (2000). Defining quality of care. *Social Science and Medicine, 51*, 1611–1625.

Coddington, D. C., Fischer, E. A., & Moore, K. D. (2001). *Strategies for the new health care marketplace.* San Francisco: Jossey-Bass.

Davidson, P., Cockburn, J., Daly, J., & Sanson, R. (2004). Patient-centered needs assessment: Rationale for a psychometric measure for assessing needs in heart failure. *Journal of Cardiovascular Nursing, 19* (3), 164–171.

Fielden, J. M., Scott, S., & Horne, J. G. (2003). An investigation of patient satisfaction following discharge after total hip replacement surgery. *Orthopaedic Nursing, 22* (6), 429–436.

Hudak, P. L., Hogg-Johnson, S., Bombardier, C., McKeever, P. D., & Wright, J. G. (2004). Testing a new theory of patient satisfaction with treatment outcome. *Medical Care, 42* (8), 726–739.

Hughes, S. (2003). Promoting independence: The nurse as coach. *Nursing Standard, 18* (10), 42–44.

Jennings, B. M., & Loan, L. A. (1999). Patient satisfaction and loyalty among military health care beneficiaries enrolled in a managed care program. *Journal of Nursing Administration, 29* (11), 47–55.

Jones, W. J. (2000). The "business"—or "public service"—of healthcare. *Journal of Healthcare Management, 45* (5), 290–293.

Kizer, K. W. (2001). Establishing health care performance standards in an era of consumerism. *Journal of the American Medical Association, 286* (10), 1213–1217.

Mallory, T. H. (2003). Future practice risks: Obstacles with opportunities. *Clinical Orthopaedics and Related Research, 407*, 74–78.

McLoughlin, V., & Leatherman, S. (2003). Quality or financing: What drives design of the health care system? *Quality and Safety in Health Care, 12*, 136–142.

Scandlen, G. (2004). Commentary: How consumer-driven healthcare evolves in a dynamic market. *Health Services Research, 39* (4), 1113–1118.

Shelton, P. J. (2000). *Measuring and improving patient satisfaction.* Gaithersburg, MD: Aspen Publishers.

Walsh, P. (2003). We must accept that health care is a risky business. *British Medical Journal, 326*, 1333–1334.

Williams, T. (2002). Patient empowerment and ethical decision making: The patient/ partner and the right to act. *Dimensions of Critical Care Nursing, 21* (3), 100–104.

Woodring, S., Polomano, R. C., Haagen, B. F., Haack, M. M., Nunn, R. R., Miller, G. L., et al. (2004). Development and testing of patient satisfaction measures for inpatient psychiatry care. *Journal of Nursing Care Quality, 19* (2), 137–148.

Wright, J., Williams, R., & Wilkinson, J. R. (1998). Health needs assessment: Development and importance of health needs assessment. *British Medical Journal, 316,* 1310–1313.

CHAPTER 9

Visioning and Strategic Planning

Anne M. Barker

*To create and communicate a shared compelling vision
of the future along with developing a strategic plan for action
to achieve that vision for the clinical unit.*

──────── CHAPTER QUESTIONS ────────

1. Why is having a vision for the clinical unit an important leadership competency?
2. What process can be used to develop a vision for the clinical unit?
3. As a clinical leader, what should I know about the organization's strategic plan?
4. What is my role in leading the clinical unit in implementing strategic initiatives and objectives?

INTRODUCTION

In this chapter we discuss the second leadership role competency, which has two components, visioning and strategic planning. We look at these from the perspective of the entire organization to provide you with the "big picture" of these leadership responsibilities; however, the emphasis is on these competencies as they relate to your role and expectations as a clinical leader.

The foundation stone of a health care organization's success is visionary leadership, yet in many organizations visions are simply written statements that are not translated into best practices, values, and work processes to achieve goals (Yearout, Miles, & Koonce, 2001). There is a distinction between having a vision and being a visionary organization or unit. It is the latter that is the goal. This chapter provides you with knowledge and tools to enhance your visionary leadership competency.

MISSION AND VISIONS

Most, if not all, health care organizations have a mission that is formally stated in a written document that describes the reason for the organization's existence. Table 9.1 gives a sample mission statement for a hypothetical medical center. As in this example, mission statements generally describe the client population served by the organization and the services provided to this population. Unique features of the organization, such as its religious affiliation, specialized services, research and/or educational purposes, and relationship in a health care system are usually mentioned as well.

Similarly, almost all health care organizations have a vision statement that exists to guide and direct behaviors and decisions for everyone in the organization. Table 9.1 also gives a sample vision statement for the same hypothetical organization as the mission statement. As a clinical manager, you should

---

Table 9.1   Sample Mission and Vision Statements

Sample Mission Statement
The mission of Community Medical Center (CMC) is to care for patients in the greater community. It is a private, not for profit medical center and is part of the Elay Health System. The Medical Center provides a wide variety of primary, secondary, and tertiary services including the only trauma facility in the county. Additionally, a full range of medical and surgical services are offered. Pediatric and obstetric services are available, including a regional neonatal intensive care unit.

Sample Vision Statement
Community Medical Center (CMC) provides high-quality, ethical, health care in response to the needs of the community it serves. The Center commits to excellence by providing competent, respectful health care in a well-organized innovative system.

CMC endorses and encourages a continuous quality improvement, problem-solving approach, which emphasizes evidenced-based practice and analysis of systems and processes. CMC actively involves those persons and groups who are most involved with an issue. This teamwork-type approach promotes cross discipline, cross departmental, and cross divisional communication/collaboration where the overall mission and vision of the hospital take precedence in determining appropriate solutions.

CMC strives toward high patient and family satisfaction with both the outcomes of our care and the quality of our relationship with them. Because of this, we are the provider of choice in the community.

Staff members respect each other and take pride in their work and in the knowledge that they are making a difference in the lives of our patients.

Sample Clinical Unit Vision Statement
It is our goal to be the best surgical clinical unit in the county. As we use the term "best," we mean outperforming other similar units in patient and family satisfaction, having a positive reputation with the physicians and other members of the team with whom we work, having optimum patient outcomes including patient safety, and being an attractive place to work.

be aware of how the overall mission and organizational vision were developed, how they are communicated, and their importance to the success of the entire organization.

Clinical unit vision statements have not been universally adopted, but we believe they are important for the success of your unit. As a clinical unit leader you should have a written vision statement for your clinical unit that is consistent with the overall organizational vision, but is more specific to the clients and staff of your unit. This vision should then guide your unit practices and systems. The challenge for you is to provide visionary leadership for your unit to become a visionary microsystem. Table 9.1 also gives a clinical unit vision statement.

Generally, when we use the term vision in this chapter, we are referring to both organizational vision and unit vision, because their purpose and importance are the same. A vision is an image of a possible and desirable future state for the organization or unit. It must be realistic, attainable, credible, challenging, and attractive to the employees. A vision statement should reflect the core purpose of the organization/unit and demonstrate its impact on society as a whole, appealing to the values, motivation, and imagination of the staff.

The Functions of Organizational Vision

The most important function of the vision is to energize people to act in a way that is consistent with unit goals, to be innovative and to change, leading to success and excellence. Visions create a culture of commitment to values and success and provide meaning to the people in the organization.

Organizational Alignment, Commitment, and Meaning

When done correctly, the vision creates a culture of commitment by aligning and connecting diverse members of the health care team through commitment to a shared value system and future goals, giving meaning and purpose to one's work. Kiefer (1986, p. 91) describes alignment as a situation in which the members of the team operate as a whole. At the same time, individual team members can be true to themselves, as well as to the organization/unit. They are willing and able to commit to the purpose and vision, and their work provides them with personal meaning and unity with other members of the team.

Performance and Goals

Transformational leaders inspire followers to perform beyond expectation. The vision is the foundation upon which this occurs by providing a stimulus toward excellence through goal setting and defining expectations that challenge staff to stretch and reach. Visionary organizations have what are called "big, hairy, audacious goals" or BHAG's (Yearout, Miles, & Koonce, 2001). The focus is changed from a system of control in which performance is motivated through formal reward and punishment mechanisms to goal attainment.

Change

Another important function of vision is its use as a general guideline and roadmap for change. Simply put, if employees are committed to the vision and values of the organization and if the change is consistent with the vision, they are more likely to be adaptable and less resistant to changes, often initiating changes themselves. In Chapter 5 we recommended that you have a vision for specific change that you wish to make. This vision serves the same purposes as the overall organizational vision or unit vision.

Decision Making

Another important function of the vision is to help people make decisions and resolve conflicts, empowering staff to act. All decisions, big and small, should be consistent with the overall vision and direction that the organization/unit is headed. With a clear vision, it becomes much easier for everyone to make decisions without needing permission and approval from others.

Developing a Unit-Level Vision: The Role of the Clinical Leader

Developing a vision for the clinical unit is a dynamic process that should involve all the members of the unit's team. We suggest you form a core group of staff that represents everyone on the unit to develop the vision. This group should then reach out to all stakeholders for input. This is an activity that you should personally lead and not delegate to others as it is a core transformational leadership strategy.

A useful technique to begin this process is to engage in a visioning exercise. Staff should be asked to close their eyes and spend some time dreaming about how they see the unit functioning in a year. Each person then writes a brief statement of that vision.

There are two important reasons for doing this. Dreaming and sharing one's dream is a very intimate process in which staff generally does not engage. It can build the team and make meaningful connections (Senge, 1990). Second, these visions can be analyzed for commonalities and differences and become the framework for further work and refinement.

Yearout, Miles, and Koonce (2001) suggest several strategies for developing a vision:

- Allow sufficient time. Your goal is to have everyone commit to the vision, so everyone must feel he or she had a voice. The process takes time so that it is not cynically viewed as another management exercise.

- Emphasize criticality. Staff needs to understand that visioning is critical to the success of your unit and client outcomes.
- Engage discussion and arrive at consensus. The team should keep focused on the task while allowing for a free exchange of opposing ideas. Your role will be to mediate conflict to allow consensus to evolve.
- Make it relevant. Although this seems obvious, the statement must be relevant to the work that your unit does, authentic in what values it espouses, and clear and simple in its call to action.

Bennis and Nanus (1985, p. 102) provide guidance to make sure that you engage in a full consideration of issues in order to develop a vision. They suggest the clinical leader and the guiding team need the skills of foresight, world-view, hindsight, depth perception, peripheral vision, and revision. Each of these skills is defined below. Based on these aspects, Table 9.2 provides a set of questions you can distribute to your team members as you begin the visioning process.

Foresight

Although this seems obvious, the vision statement must take into account the future and be consistent with the mission. A basic question is, "Why are we in business and what business should we be in for the future?"

Although knowing the future is almost impossible to predict, the clinical leader and the team need to be aware of the trends, issues, and predictions for the future of health care. This means keeping up with the professional literature and attending meetings, both internally and externally.

Worldview

Having a worldview is similar to foresight. It means having a broad understanding of societal trends and issues both locally and globally. Yearout, Miles, and Koonce (2001) propose what they call a business climate model to approach these questions. They suggest you consider technology, economics, political, and customer factors.

Hindsight

Understanding the history of the organization is vital in not only developing a vision statement but in becoming a visionary unit. The clinical leader and vision team should understand and appreciate the traditions of the organization as a whole and the clinical unit specifically, the organizational culture, and the relationship of the organization to the community over time.

Table 9.2   Questions for Developing the Clinical Unit Vision Statement

Foresight

- Why are we in business?
- What are the trends in health care that impact the unit now or are expected to impact the unit in the future?
- What are the demographics regarding the future workforce and what are the implications for our unit?
- What are the strengths of the staff and of our unit?
- Who are our clients and what do they expect from us?

Worldview

- What societal trends, both local and global, will impact health care and the clinical professions? (Consider technology, economics, political, and customer factors.)

Hindsight

- What is the current mission and vision of the organization? Has it changed recently or is it likely to change in the future?
- What is the history of the organization and our unit and how does this affect who we are?

Depth Perception

- What resources in terms of people, money, and space are available to us?
- What is the match between the internal strength of the organization/unit and the needs of the community?
- What other stakeholders need to be brought into this process?
- How do the current systems of organization and management, such as the care delivery system, information system, and financial management system, affect our unit and its future?

Peripheral Vision

- Who are our competitors and what are their strengths and weaknesses?

Revision

- How well has the vision served us over the last year?
- Have we had to make decisions that were inconsistent with the vision? Why?
- What has happened in the external environment that affects our vision?

Depth Perception

Depth perception suggests that the clinical leader and vision team consider the "whole picture" of the organization. This includes consideration of all employees on the team, the population and community served, other stakeholders, and the current systems of organization and management, such as the care delivery system, information systems, and financial management systems.

Peripheral Vision

This skill involves an understanding of competitors both within the organization and outside the organization.

Revision

After the vision statement has been developed, you should evaluate and review the statement periodically to see how it is helping, or not, the unit be successful. It also requires that the clinical leader continually assess the external environment for changes that impact on the organization department and the vision.

The Vision Statement

The vision statement for your clinical unit should have two dimensions. First, it should focus on the client care management systems and outcomes. The second dimension should focus on the staff and their role in providing client services in an environment that is satisfying and meaningful. Logically, the vision at the unit level must be consistent with the overall vision and mission of the entire organization.

Complexity science further informs the visioning process and need for a vision. However, complexity science tells us that the world and organizations are unknowable and unpredictable, certainly a paradox. The answer is to have a vision in which strategies are not predetermined. As an example, having and implementing a vision of "providing world-class cancer care to individuals in the community" provides strategic direction and allows creative approaches. In contrast having and implementing a vision of providing world-class care to an increased market share of 10 percent more patients in the community to increase revenues by x dollars while maintaining the same expenses, limits the direction and stifles creativity.

Living the Vision

The hardest part of becoming a visionary unit is to live the vision once it is developed. You must communicate the vision widely and often and embed it in virtually all activities. Visionary leaders use metaphors and analogies to express the vision or short jingles or "sound bites." One clinical unit whose vision entailed becoming self staffed played on the theme of floating, "You won't be left up the creek without a paddle!" became a funny refrain that was shared among the staff.

It is difficult to behave consistently and to make decisions based on the unit vision. As a visionary leader you must be able to explain an action or change based on how it moves forward the vision. In times of crises or when an action that is inconsistent with the vision must be taken, it must be honestly and openly discussed and explained. This may also present a need to revisit the vision itself. If not, discontent will set in and undermine the vision.

STRATEGIC PLANNING

The second component of the competency is to determine specific strategies based on the vision. Strategic planning is most often thought of as an organizational effort led by the chief executive officer. However, in some organizations departments and units also have strategic plans. As a clinical leader, you may or may not have direct input into the overall strategic plan or you may have indirect input in it through your boss. Whatever your role, it is important to understand how a strategic plan is developed. Further, since the tactics of the strategic plan happen at the unit level where the providers and the clients interact, it is impossible for an organization to have a useful strategic plan unless everyone in the organization is aware of and working toward the plan.

After reading this section, you may decide to have a strategic plan for your unit and can use this information to develop a plan for your unit. We first describe the process of preparing a strategic plan and then discuss the implications of this plan on your role as a clinical leader.

Strategic Planning Committees

Organizations vary widely as to who develops the strategic plan but generally it occurs in one of three ways, with variations of each, depending on the leadership style of the chief executive officer and the size of the organization. At one end of the continuum, a department charged with the responsibility of strategic planning for the organization may be the primary developer and writer of the plan. A more inclusive approach is that the plan may be developed by a committee composed primarily of people at the executive level of the organization. At the other end of the spectrum would be a strategic planning committee that is widely representative of all of the staff in the organization.

Steps in Strategic Planning

For our purposes we are talking about the overall organization's strategic plan, but if you choose to develop a strategic plan for your unit you can follow this approach as well. The following steps are usually followed when developing or revising a strategic plan:

1. Scan the internal environment.
2. Conduct a scan of the external environment.
3. Conduct a SWOT (strengths, weaknesses, opportunities, threats) analysis.
4. Create or revise the vision, if needed.
5. Develop strategic initiatives.
6. Implement strategic plans.
7. Evaluate the results.

Internal Scan

The strategic planning process begins with looking at the organizational mission, value statement, and vision. Before moving forward the organization must have a clear understanding of what business it is in and to whom they provide services.

External Environmental Scan

The next step is a scan of the external environment. In completing the scan of the external environment, consideration is given to societal values, the competition, workforce supply and demand, the customers, political issues and trends, other stakeholders, the economy, changing technology, demands from payers, regulators, accreditors, and so forth.

SWOT Analysis

Next, complete a SWOT analysis for the organization. This is an analysis of the organization's strengths, weaknesses, opportunities, and threats.

To assess organizational strengths, review the organization's competitive advantage, what the organization does well, what resources the organization has access to, the strengths and skills of the employees, successes it has had in the past to build on, capital assets, the financial health of the organization (or not), the reputation of the organization in the community, and so forth.

Similarly, the strategic planning group will look at the organization's weaknesses and consider what the competition does better than your organization, what needs be improved in the organization, what resources are not available, technological issues, financial insufficiencies, reputation in the community, and deficiencies among the staff in regard to specific skills.

Next, opportunities and threats are considered. These are derived from the scan of the external environment matched to the strengths and weaknesses of the organization. In other words, some external factors will provide opportunities for the organization that match its strengths, and other external factors will be threats to the organization where the organization is weak.

Create or Revise the Vision

Once the scan of the internal and external environment and the SWOT analysis are completed, it may be necessary to revise the mission statement. Often mission statements remain constant for many years but completing the first three steps of the strategic planning process provides an opportunity to review and affirm the mission. Likewise, it may be necessary to create a vision statement if one does not exist or revise an existing one. The steps and process outlined in the first section of this chapter would then be taken.

Strategic Initiatives and Objectives

In this step the planning group brings together all the above elements to determine strategic initiatives, which are generally broad statements. These then have multiple short-term objectives (or goals) that need to be completed to meet the overarching initiative. Table 9.3 is an extract from a strategic plan for a community hospital.

Implement the Plans

As a clinical manager, this is generally where you first become involved in the strategic planning process. You may be asked to develop and meet objectives that contribute to the achievement of the organization's strategic plan.

Table 9.3   Sample Strategic Initiatives and Objectives

Strategic Initiative
To develop and maintain an attractive and appropriately equipped physical plant that is ideally suited to our role and mission as a community hospital.

Strategic Objectives
1. Engage the services of an architectural firm to assess the physical plant and equipment and develop a five-year master plan.
2. Conduct an assessment of equipment to see what needs to be replaced or upgraded.
3. Improve signage throughout the building.
4. Review the possible impact or implications of pending changes in the Centers for Medicare and Medicaid Life Safety Code Requirements.
5. Survey staff and patients regarding the cleanliness of the facility and take appropriate action.

You can refer to the change model in Chapter 5 to set forth a plan for implementing these objectives.

Evaluate Progress

The final step is evaluating progress at some predetermined time and measuring successes. At this point the plan can be revised based on changes in the external environment and progress or lack of progress on specific initiatives.

Role of the Clinical Leader

Whether or not you have had input into the organizational strategic plan, you still have responsibility for helping the organization meet its objectives. In fact, looking at the clinical unit as a microsystem it is where the strategic plan either succeeds or fails.

Your role is to:

- Read the strategic plan.
- Extract from the plan those initiatives and objectives that are pertinent to your unit.
- Share these with your staff and help them to make meaning.
- Use the change model in Chapter 5 to implement processes to achieve goals.
- Reward and recognize successes.

One final role should be highlighted. You are the spokesperson for your clinical unit. You should tell your story to others outside your clinical unit when you have successes and share how your staff has contributed to the overall strategic plan and to the ultimate success of the organization.

SCENARIO

Sarah is the new nurse manager of a general medical unit in a 350-bed urban hospital. Another hospital in the same city is a major competitor. The two hospitals share medical staff from a local university, have the same group of private physicians, and compete for employees from the same workforce pool.

Sarah has had previous experience as a nurse manager in another state. When being interviewed for the job, she was informed that the unit needed a strong leader who could increase staff morale and decrease vacancy rates and staff turnover. She learned that the patient satisfaction scores for the unit consistently fell below both national and institutional scores and admitting physicians preferred to send their patients to the competitor hospital when admitted for general medicine.

Sarah assesses the situation and believes that she first needs to engage the staff in the development of a vision statement for the clinical unit. To do this, she forms a task force, headed by herself, representing nurses, unlicensed associates, and secretaries from all three shifts and members of the interdisciplinary team who are assigned to the unit including a housekeeper, dietitian, social worker, attending physician, and pharmacist.

At the first meeting of the task force, she asked each of the members to participate in a visioning exercise. She asked them to close their eyes and think about how they would like to see the unit one year from now. Then she asked them to write what they envisioned. All the members then shared their vision and Sarah compiled the results. The major themes that emerged were:

- General medicine should be viewed with respect—not as an unpleasant and unsatisfying work.
- Since over 80 percent of the patients coming to the unit were diagnosed with a comorbidity of diabetes and heart failure, the staff should be experts not generalists in these two disease entities.
- The health care team should work together cohesively.
- People should have fun and enjoy what they do when they come to work.
- Patients should experience excellent outcomes in a safe environment.
- Patients should be highly satisfied with their care, so that the clinical unit would become their unit of choice when needing to be hospitalized or when referring others.
- Admitting physicians would prefer to admit their patients to this unit rather than to the competitor's.

From this work, the team developed the following vision statement:

The staff on Nine West is committed to contributing to an environment in which people are proud to work, are committed to their work, and have fun. The staff works together collaboratively and cohesively to realize the goals of the clinical unit. All employees on the unit will have the opportunity to contribute to the success of the unit in an environment that fosters growth and learning. The staff respects each other and treats each other fairly.

Our clients will receive world-class care based on evidence and professional standards. We will be the provider of choice for our subpopulation of patients and physicians.

SCENARIO ANALYSIS

Visioning is one of the premier strategies for the transformational leader. For this reason, Sarah chose to lead this effort herself. However, Sarah's ongoing task will to be to provide visionary leadership for the clinical unit. Using the new vision statement, Sarah will have to build trust, make decisions, and take action based on the vision. The vision statement itself sets high expectations for the staff and, if achieved, will be one strategy for increasing staff self-esteem.

In this scenario the clinical leader used at least three principles of complexity science: *cultivating relationships, taking small steps,* and *making sense and meaning.* By setting up the vision team from diverse members of the staff, she put together individuals who generally only interact around specific patient care and daily operations. These individuals had to interact at a deeper, more meaningful level as they dreamt about and planned the future together. Sarah also used the complexity science principle of sense making. The act of developing a vision is an act of discovery and understanding what is happening and why it is happening. Further, as a new manager Sarah was presented with an overwhelming task of increasing patient and staff satisfaction. Sarah started with a small step, developing the vision, rather than writing a sophisticated long-term plan.

In this scenario Sarah fulfilled the Leadership IQ roles of *connector* and *synergizer.* She connected with staff and she designed a system and set forth a task to have others connect as well. As synergizer, she empowered the staff to take control of the future.

APPLICATION EXERCISES

1. Review your organization's mission and vision statements.
2. If you do not have a vision for your unit, form a vision team and use Table 9.2 to begin discussion. Have the team read this chapter of the book.

REFERENCES

Bennis, W., & Nanus, B. (1985). *Leaders: Strategies for taking charge.* New York: Harper & Row.

Kiefer, C. (1986). Leadership in metanoic organizations. In J. D. Adams (ed.) *Transforming leadership: From vision to results.* Alexandria, VA: Miles River Press.

Senge, P. (1990). *The fifth discipline.* New York: Doubleday.

Yearout, S., Miles, G., & Koonce, R. H. (2001). Multi-level visioning. *Training and Development, 55* (3).

CHAPTER 10

Managing Care Across the Continuum

Dori Taylor Sullivan

To foster systems to coordinate care across health care settings to promote optimal client outcomes and cost-effective, resource-efficient care.

CHAPTER QUESTIONS

1. How much and in what ways are managed care strategies influencing care within my region?
2. How do changing patterns in care for various client populations relate to my areas?
3. What model(s) of case management and/or disease management exist in my organization or in significant payer groups?
4. To what extent are clinical practice guidelines or pathways influencing care in my organization and am I appropriately involved in that process?
5. What are the key role relationships between case managers and other health care providers and service areas and how could I enhance those relationships to better serve clients?

INTRODUCTION

Changes in the health care system including technology, concerns regarding increasing costs of care, and client preferences have led to a dramatic shift in where numerous popular procedures and treatments are performed. Techniques like minimally invasive and laparoscopic surgery have shortened recovery times and may even be done in ambulatory surgery settings, requiring no overnight hospital stays. Because hospitals remain the most costly of health care settings, moving the location of care delivery to less intensive settings can reduce care costs significantly. The question remains, though, as to which procedures and treatments require the resources of an acute care hospital setting to assure proper patient safety. Lastly, most people would prefer to have care within their home or community, and this factor also supports the delivery of care in other than hospital locations whenever reasonable to do so.

To meet this increasing demand, various types of health care organizations have proliferated and expanded. There are now freestanding surgical centers, and many physicians perform procedures in their offices that just a few years ago required hospital stays. Skilled nursing facilities or nursing homes have opened units for more acutely ill patients and have expanded the skills and treatments provided in addition to creating specialty care units for short-term rehabilitation, memory loss and dementia, and other patient groups with special needs. Assisted-living facilities and life care communities with multiple levels of health services are appearing all over the country to serve older Americans. Home care agencies have also expanded their services, skills, hours, and staffing to meet community needs. And of course, there are family primary care and the spectrum of specialty physician practices also seeing patients for various complaints and diagnoses.

The proliferation of settings and services has created new demands for coordinating care to obtain best outcomes, preventing harm through duplication or conflicting therapies, and reducing overuse of health care services that increase costs. When we consider these factors with the general aging of the population, we are seeing more fragile clients with multiple chronic diseases. So when a chronically ill patient of seventy presents to a health care facility, it is likely that the acute problem will need to be addressed with consideration of existing and perhaps exacerbated chronic conditions.

This chapter describes the various roles used to coordinate and manage care within and across settings with specific attention to case managers and the relatively new approach of disease management. Some of the major functions handled by case and/or disease management specialists include discharge planning, utilization review, communication with payers, clinical guidelines, quality indicator measurement, and quality improvement (QI) activities. Most important, we examine the key relationships among case or disease management and clinical leaders in your areas. Depending on your responsibilities, you may have direct or indirect involvement with coordinators of care. Whatever the nature of the interactions, these coordinators are influencing your unit in a positive or negative way. If you provide direct services to patients, the case manager will want to assure that the care is justifiable, timely, and covered by that patient's insurer. If, for example, you work in the laboratory and never see patients, a change in physician practice or clinical guidelines could result in a significant increase or decrease in a certain type of test that is performed. As a clinical leader you have a great opportunity to enhance both the quality and the cost of care through innovative approaches to delivering and coordinating care.

THE LANGUAGE OF MANAGING CARE

Let's begin by clarifying some of the language related to the management and coordination of care. The term *managed care* can refer to either an organization or a process.

Considering the reference to an organization, when *managed care* is used we tend to think of a health maintenance organization (HMO) or managed care company like an insurance group. In this context, managed care may be defined as "a means of providing health care services within a network of health care providers. The central concept is coordination of all health care services for an individual" (Baker & Baker, 2004, p. 199). The coordination aspect refers to authorizing the care and assuring that the care is provided according to agreed-upon standards. Some managed care plans require a gatekeeper, often a primary care provider or internist, who must preapprove or make the referral to a specialist. The network of providers may be large in number or relatively restricted. Some plans make provisions for out of network services with a higher cost to patients, while others do not allow out of network coverage.

In a traditional HMO virtually all care is provided by the organization's medical providers and services while members pay a designated amount per month whether they use services or not. At the other end of the spectrum is the fee for service model, with a wide choice of physicians and health care organizations and little restriction on what services are sought. Medicare patients may be in an HMO or more of a fee for service structure, depending on their geographical location and choice of provider. Most state Medicaid plans now require managed care enrollment.

As a clinical leader, it is crucial that you have a sense of who the major purchasers or payers of your services are and to what extent they are using managed care principles in the agreements in place. The more managed care types of plans that exist, the more requirements or restrictions there will likely be for clients and for you as a provider. You also need to be familiar with the specific requirements and how much reimbursement is provided for each type of patient or service. We discuss this in detail in Chapter 15 on financial outcomes.

Managing care in the general sense reflects the goal of all health care providers involved in an individual's care to work in an effective and coordinated fashion to share information, establish priorities for treatment while at the same time considering other conditions and patient preferences, to achieve desired outcomes. Few patients would say they do not want their care coordinated or managed using this definition.

Now the question is, "How does that management of care or coordination happen?"

CASE MANAGEMENT

Case management (CM) has evolved to mean many things, depending on the setting where practiced, the model of care management developed, and the related goals established for the CM role. Case management has been defined by the Case Management Society of America (CMSA) as "a collaborative process of assessment, planning, facilitation and advocacy for options and services to meet an individual's health needs through communication and available resources to promote quality cost-effective outcomes" (CMSA, 2005).

Case managers (CMs) may be found in hospitals, insurance or managed care companies, physician practices, home care agencies, and other settings. The true goals of the organization for its CM program may include medical utilization management, cost reduction, decreasing variation in the care across patient populations, and overall improvement of quality and outcomes (see Table 10.1). The multitude of settings and goals for CM practice has created confusion about what a CM really is.

The Case Manager Role

The CM role has generally centered on transitioning patients from more costly services to less intensive and less costly services and/or settings. Effective CM in most settings involves the following activities:

- Identification of high risk or complex patients who require CM.
- Initial and ongoing assessments to determine individual needs and preferences and to serve as a patient advocate.
- Development of an individual plan of care with clinical guidelines or pathways as the foundation, considering realistic desired outcomes and financial implications.
- Planning for discharge setting and services.
- Communication with insurers or payers regarding benefits, current status, and alternatives for care across settings.
- Coordinating treatments and services within the care setting.
- Evaluation of progress and revision of the individual plan of care based on reassessments.
- Participation in quality and program evaluation processes.
- Consideration of ethical, legal, and regulatory issues and standards (Powell, 2000; Radzwill, 2002).

Case managers typically oversee all professional services as the coordinator of care. Most CMs are registered nurses; however, other professionals such

Table 10.1   Sample Case Manager Position Description

Position:	CASE MANAGER
Department:	Quality and Care Coordination
Education:	BSN required, Master's Degree preferred in related area plus current RN license
Experience:	Two years of recent acute care practice

Position Summary:

Performs care coordination, utilization management, and discharge planning activities across the continuum of care in collaboration with physicians and other health care professionals. Maintains ongoing communication with appropriate internal and external parties regarding individual patients' care, authorizations, progress, and changes. Participates in development, data collection, analysis, and improvement of evidence-based clinical guidelines, care processes, and quality outcomes.

Responsibilities:

Care Coordination (30%)

- Assess high-risk patients, determine needs, formulate specific plans, and evaluate results.
- Monitor progress of pathway/plan of care and facilitate necessary discussions with health team members.
- Collaborate with and provide information to patients, families, physicians, and staff about patient needs/progress.

Utilization Management (30%)

- Perform preadmission, admission, and concurrent utilization management reviews using guidelines and other information to determine appropriate level of care.
- Communicate with physicians and others to resolve utilization and systems' issues interfering with patient care.
- Communicate with insurance companies, HMOs, and other payers regarding patient status, needs, and progress.
- Analyze utilization reports for assigned areas and provide this information to clinical leaders for each area.

Discharge Planning (20%)

- Develop a comprehensive plan for discharge according to guidelines, standards, and patient needs/preferences.
- Consult with other departments and agencies to provide seamless transitions to home or another facility.

Quality Improvement (20%)

- Participate in the development of clinical guidelines.
- Promote data-driven improvement activities to enhance outcomes.

as physical therapists and social workers may be CMs depending on the needs of the patient populations served. Depending on your role as a clinical leader, some of your staff may be CMs, or they may work collaboratively with CMs to provide comprehensive services. Or, you and your staff may need to provide information or documentation to external CMs for authorization of service or on a patient's behalf. Understanding the role and functions of the CM should promote open communication and problem-solving activities to best serve the client.

Case Management Outcomes

The CM process has been effectively used in acute care, outpatient, home care, and other settings with diverse client groups and health care needs. Substantial literature supports that CM has been successful in improving quality and reducing costs through effective use of institutional resources and close monitoring of care needs and level of service required (Cudney, 2002; Ramsey, Ormsby, & Marsh, 2001). In hospitals this has usually translated into shorter lengths of stay (LOS), a strong predictor of costs of a hospitalization. Cudney (2002) also noted that CM is a key factor in increasing quality of care, patient satisfaction, compliance, and quality of life.

Powell (2000, pp. 55–59) suggested a host of CM outcomes of interest related to quality of care, collaboration, fiscal responsibilities, patient advocacy, outpatient management, and professional nursing practice. When performed well, CM should improve the quality of care and patient satisfaction while reducing risks and adverse events, promote physician satisfaction and team collaboration, reduce costs for delays and unnecessary treatments, support and educate the patient and family while advocating for them, anticipate and plan for discharge needs, and enhance the professional practice of nursing and other health disciplines.

Harrison, Nolin, and Suero (2004) conducted a study to look at the effect of case management on hospitals in the United States. They determined that from an operating performance perspective, hospitals with a case management program had higher occupancy rates and lower operating expenses per discharge. Hospitals with case management programs tended to be larger with more services and higher presence of managed care versus fee for service. They also tended to be located in areas with fewer older people and with higher per capita incomes. A conclusion of the study was that hospitals in markets with more HMO penetration were using case management programs to improve efficiency and compete for HMO business. When successful in these two goals, the contribution of CMs to hospital and other health care organization success is significant.

DISEASE MANAGEMENT

The concept of disease management is a relatively recent phenomenon that has grown popular as dissatisfaction with restricted access to care has grown. Disease management is considered as a more sophisticated and humanistic approach that can both enhance health care services and patient outcomes while potentially reducing costs and encouraging the wise use of resources.

What Is Disease Management?

According to the Disease Management Association of America (DMAA), disease management (DM) is "a system of coordinated health care interventions and communications for populations with conditions in which patient self-care efforts are significant" (DMAA, 2005). The DMAA further states that a full service DM program must include six components:

- Population identification processes
- Evidence-based practice guidelines
- Collaborative practice models to include physician and support-service providers
- Patient self-management education (may include primary prevention, behavior modification programs, and compliance/surveillance)
- Process and outcomes measurement, evaluation, and management
- Routine reporting/feedback loop (may include communication with the patient, physician, health plan and ancillary providers, and practice profiling)

Disease management is also said to support practitioner/patient relationships; emphasize prevention of exacerbations and complication through evidence-based guidelines and patient empowerment strategies; and evaluate clinical, humanistic, and economic outcomes on an ongoing basis with the goal of improving overall health.

As with case managers, DM specialists may be employed by clinical agencies, insurance companies and managed care organizations, or other entities with an interest in promoting the health of their members or clients. As with CM, the true objectives and focus of DM varies with who funds the program.

What the Research Says About Disease Management

A sizable study by Fireman, Bartlett, and Selby (2004) asked whether disease management can reduce health care costs by improving quality. They reported that in 2000 a survey of 45 health plans revealed that more than half had a DM program in place. The study assessed cost and quality outcomes for adults with four common conditions: coronary artery disease, heart failure, diabetes, and asthma. Programs for DM of these conditions had been developed and implemented. The researchers analyzed seven years of data and found that many of the quality indicators showed positive changes; however, costs also were higher. The overall conclusion was that while costs might have increased more without DM, the only way DM would save money was if the treatments themselves were less costly. In a critique of this study (Crosson & Madvig, 2004), other experts were complimentary of the study but said that the cost calculation methodology was very conservative, and in fact, DM may well have saved money. Clearly, more studies are needed in this area.

A COMBINED CASE AND DISEASE MANAGEMENT MODEL

It may make sense to create a combined case and disease management model to better integrate these functions in a seamless care management process that promotes optimal client outcomes (Radzwill, 2002).

Taken together, CM and DM create a comprehensive approach to learning more about higher risk populations, especially those with common chronic conditions. This knowledge can then be used to identify at risk patients and build clinical guidelines that encompass the entire continuum of care. Approached this way, it is important to think of the entire course of an illness rather than just the hospital or home care portion of the treatment. Perhaps most important, embracing a combined model requires a commitment to prevention and education as much as to diagnosis and treatment—a major paradigm shift even though it has been discussed for a long time. Some experts refer to this combined model as *care management.*

Case or disease managers must have extensive knowledge of insurance types and plans that cover their clients as well as solid working knowledge of utilization management skills and techniques. Utilization management (UM) is a structured process using established criteria to determine and document medical necessity of treatment, appropriate level of care, and timing of discharge. A variety of UM activities occur in different phases of care delivery, including preadmission review or certification, concurrent review for continuing stay, and retrospective reviews. Today, telephone reviews along with electronic communications are the methods of choice to save health care personnel and payer time.

Important Tools Supporting Case and Disease Management

The success of CM and DM depends on developing an organizational infrastructure to support them. This infrastructure should include defining and communicating clear objectives, methodology for developing clinical guidelines that are evidence based and endorsed by involved health providers, and user friendly information technology (IT) systems and support. The importance of IT cannot be overstated, for without obtaining data, the evaluation of quality, performance, and outcomes will be elusive. In Chapter 11 we discuss how to create a quality of culture, including the specifics of evidence-based practice and guidelines, and principles for effective IT systems. Here we highlight how evidence-based clinical pathways or guidelines facilitate the CM and DM processes as well as providing an overview of outcomes assessment.

Evidence-Based Clinical Pathways

One of the best contributions of the focus on quality and performance measurement is recognizing that many health disciplines play a role in promoting client health or recovery. The best plans of care include specifics regarding the actions each health care provider is expected to take at what point in time, based on knowledge of predicted responses, resulting in a multidisciplinary plan of care. This knowledge is derived from both formal education and clinical experience. Over time the phrase *clinical* or *critical* pathway (CP) has come to mean a multidisciplinary approach to caring for different patient groups that contains the most important actions and timelines (see Table 10.2).

In the example of a patient who experienced an acute myocardial infarction, the CP would cover assessment expectations, lab work and parameters, activity progression, diet, patient education, and rehabilitation. Examples of CPs are available in books, journals, and on the Internet. These sources are a good place to start, but two other activities are needed. First, the clinicians who provide the care must be actively engaged and endorse the guidelines developed for a particular area or institution. Without this buy-in, the guidelines may look wonderful but have little impact on care. Second, a process for evaluating and incorporating new evidence or research in relevant areas ensures that the guidelines reflect current best practice. In addition to research findings, there are industry publications containing recommended standards related to levels of care or settings, amount of care (for example, length of stay or number of visits) that heavily influence payer and provider standards. Two of the most common publications are Milliman Care Guidelines (2005) and Interqual (2005).

Clinical leaders must be ready to participate and prepare their staffs for involvement in developing evidence-based CPs. Done well, this is an exciting and rewarding activity that can promote strong and positive relationships among members of the health care team. All providers of care must be familiar with the CPs, thus education of staff and accessibility to the CPs become critical enabling factors. Each organization tends to develop its own methods of

Table 10.2   Sample Clinical Pathway

Clinical Pathway: DRG # <u>209</u>	Total Knee Replacement Estimated LOS <u>3 days</u>		
	Day 1 (Surgery)	**Day 2 (POD 1)**	**Day 3 (POD 2)**
Assessment	Confirm preop X-ray		
Diagnostics	Postop X-ray		
Treatments	Postop care protocol* CPM machine CMS checks Q2h		
Medications	IVF per orders Pain med PCA/IM Anticoagulant IV antibiotic	IV > lock Pain med IM/PO Anticoagulant	IV d/c Pain med PO Anticoagulant
Activity	Bedrest	OOB per PT	OOB per PT
Nutrition		Clear liq if BS + and N/V − (AM) Reg diet (PM) I & O	Reg diet
Education	Review preop ed	Home exercise plan	Repeat home exercise plan Review meds Call for advice
Consultations		PT, HHC/ECF, Soc Svcs, DME	PT, HHC/ECF, Soc Svcs, DME
Desired Outcomes	VS stable postop Pain <3 on scale Discharge plan	OOB Pain <3 on scale Afebrile Discharge plan confirmed	Inc. activity Pain <2 States activity & ed plan Discharged per plan

* describes care for all patients after a surgical procedure

Preadmission Activities
      [   ] General education about joint replacement
      [   ] Initial assessment and education by PT
Discharge Planning Notes
      [   ] Initial assessment by RN for tentative discharge plan
Individual Considerations

Admission Date_____ Payer/Plan_____

creating CPs and systematically reviewing and updating them. Case managers and quality specialists are frequently charged with leading the process of maintaining and updating CPs.

There is an obvious connection of the CPs to CM and DM since the CPs specify the major tests and treatments that patients should receive and their expected response and progression. Case managers rely on these markers to assess where a patient is during the course of an illness. The CM also considers the guidelines established by the payer and communicates relevant information to that payer as required so that appropriate care can continue.

Managing Information to Support Care Management

Often CPs are automated to facilitate the collection of data about whether a given patient is progressing as planned or not; and if not, why and what will be done about it. In well-developed care management systems, quality indicators for care processes and patient outcomes are included as part of the CP; data related to each indicator is entered into the IT system by designated personnel.

Many comprehensive health management information systems (HMIS) use software for entering and analyzing this type of data since it has become a mainstay in health care practice. Numerous stand-alone systems for elements of the information needed, for example, CPs, are also available but may require more data entry if they cannot interface with and transfer necessary information from other institutional systems.

We should also mention the issues of data integrity and security. Data integrity refers to the accuracy of data. Mistakes may occur with the clarity of coding, the accuracy of coding, and the accuracy of data entry among others. Reasonable steps must be taken to demonstrate data integrity to have confidence in the information provided. Security of health information has always been of concern but even more so today with HIPAA requirements in full force. In addition, plans for data storage, backup, and how CM will operate should the systems malfunction are essential.

KEY RELATIONSHIPS FOR EFFECTIVE CARE MANAGEMENT

Much of what CMs and DMs do is dependent upon the quality of relationships and communication. Whether in person or on the telephone, the CM is often in the position of negotiating as she advocates for clients and for her organization. Some of the most important relationships are with physicians, nurses, allied health professionals, payers, other health care organizations and community resources like pharmacies and medical supply companies.

These relationships are presented next, noting desired outcomes and potential issues.

Physician leadership and participation in the development of CPs is one of the most important elements for success. In optimal situations, CMs and DMs work collaboratively with physicians to move patients through the health care system continuum according to the CPs to deliver effective and efficient care. Case managers can also provide specific performance information about individual physician practice patterns for use in assessment and improvement. Physicians sometimes feel overanalyzed and oversupervised given regulatory and organizational changes in recent years. The ability to create a positive partnership with physicians around enhancing care to clients through CM and DM are hallmarks of seasoned practitioners.

Similarly, CMs and DMs need supportive and collaborative relationships with nurses. Nurses provide important information related to patient needs and progress along with issues that concern them. It is desirable that the nurses identify the CM/DM as an ally in patient advocacy. Nurses and CMs/DMs have a need for regular communication with involved physicians, but for somewhat different reasons. When the relationship between nurses and CMs/DMs is not going well, nurses can feel like the CM/DM is supplanting their role as a professional nurse with primary responsibility for a patient.

Depending on the nature of the patient populations, different allied health professions are involved in their care. The CM or DM works collaboratively with these colleagues as well to check on progress, discuss issues, and consider plans for the next phase of care.

The CM is often the face or voice of a health care institution in dealing with an insurer or HMO responsible for paying for the care a member is receiving. Often this relationship is fraught with tension as payers state what benefits are covered while the CM tries to obtain what clients need. The DM approach brings the two closer together as they partner to achieve the best outcomes— for the client while considering cost perspectives. But, make no mistake, issues still occur. Developing a relationship and a level of trust with major payers serves everyone well and is the desired situation.

The relationships among health care organizations providing different levels of care are also usually through CMs and are especially crucial when a more acute setting is trying to move a patient to the appropriate level of care. Many a talented CM has been able to secure a timely and desirable placement or contract for services due to her relationship with colleagues at the receiving end. If there is trust in the assessment of client needs rather than a sense that a difficult patient is being offloaded, the transfer proceeds more smoothly.

Familiarity with community resources can contribute greatly to patient transitions by assuring that the required supplies or services will be there when needed. Whether it is a hospital bed, home oxygen, or hospice care, patient and family need the assurance that care and comfort needs will be handled.

In summary, CMs and DMs develop positive, trusting relationships with key individuals and groups while applying their expert knowledge of evidence-based quality care and payer requirements to coordinate care resulting in optimal outcomes for clients and cost effective services.

SCENARIO

Frances is the CM for an orthopedics unit in a hospital where she regularly sees patients who have had total joint replacements. There is a well-written, evidence-based CP for total knee replacement surgery patients that is supported by the regular orthopedic surgeons who practice in this institution. This CP covers the full continuum of care services because it has been shown that pre and post hospital care significantly affect some of the important patient outcomes.

Dr. Ryan is a joint replacement surgeon who joined the medical staff about two months ago. After hearing from Gary, the physical therapist, that joint replacement patients seemed to have more questions than usual about what was going to happen postoperatively, Frances reviewed a number of recent discharge records. She noticed a trend among Dr. Ryan's patients indicating that they had not made appointments with the office nurse for preoperative teaching. This teaching includes a brief video about the joint replacement procedure and an initial assessment and practice session with physical therapy. Several published studies and hospital-specific evaluations had shown that the preoperative teaching appointment contributed to decreased patient anxiety and increased compliance with postoperative activity related to rehabilitation therapy.

Frances has enjoyed a highly collaborative relationship with most of the physicians she has dealt with in her CM role. She suspects that Dr. Ryan has not been made aware of this important part of the CP, so she decides to discuss this with him. Frances selected a relatively quiet time on the unit when she and Dr. Ryan were seated working with charts.

Frances expected that Dr. Ryan would be receptive to her conversation because there had been no issues in their work together to date. She was shocked and upset when Dr. Ryan interrupted her after two sentences basically telling her to mind her own business, that his patients were within the guidelines for expected lengths of stay and that he didn't need someone watching his every move and telling him what to do. Frances stopped the conversation and decided to seek advice from Dr. Jason, one of the surgeons she knew best, so that she could pursue the matter in a constructive way.

SCENARIO ANALYSIS

Frances and Dr. Jason realized that Dr. Ryan did not seem to share the vision for a seamless continuum of care services. They also agreed that there were trust issues and probably empowerment issues operating as well, but they had no idea for the reasons behind them at this point. (A shared vision, fostering trust, and empowerment are three of the elements of a transformational leader.)

Frances considered several LIQ roles in her assessment of the situation. She wondered whether she needed to adjust her communication style in her *connector* role. From the *evaluator* perspective, she was convinced that the data strongly supported the importance of that preoperative visit. She had further assumed that Dr. Ryan was aware of this information but maybe he wasn't. The *protector* role played a part in that Frances was well aware that a very positive word of mouth communication pattern had increased their orthopedic procedures and was something the surgeons and institution wanted to build on; so anything that threatened that was of concern. Finally, Frances and Dr. Jason speculated that some of the *healer* role might be necessary since Dr. Ryan's reaction seemed out of proportion to what had been said. Perhaps he had experienced negative interactions or consequences with CMs or other roles he perceived were overseeing his work inappropriately.

As a *complex adaptive system* (CAS) embedded in numerous other CASs, Dr. Ryan was reacting and adapting to his relatively new environment. Dr. Jason and Frances agreed that it would be helpful if Dr. Jason as well as Frances tried to create collaborative relationships with Dr. Ryan. Dr. Jason had commented that Dr. Ryan had been relatively quiet during the few meetings they had attended together; he had not interacted much with anyone. Their intuition was that Dr. Ryan was not feeling comfortable in his new environment.

Taking all of the above into account, Dr. Jason invited Dr. Ryan to lunch and spent some time speaking about the nature of relationships at this institution and their pride in the outcomes achieved with this teamwork in the context of evidence-based CPs. Dr. Jason also described Frances' contributions and commitment to these achievements and how much he respected her skills. He suggested that Dr. Ryan participate in one of the informal review sessions of the CP team to get a sense of what the evaluation data was showing and how the team worked together. While no miracles were accomplished, Dr. Ryan did follow through with some of Dr. Jason's suggestions, and Frances was able to make the important points without singling Dr. Ryan out. Her strategy was to work on developing the relationship to a comfortable level before discussing his specific practice, not because he is a doctor, but because of the insights she received from applying these theories or lenses with a colleague/mentor.

APPLICATION EXERCISES

1. Thinking of the major client groups you are involved with, determine who the major payers are and to what extent clients are in some type of managed care plan.

2. Ask an appropriate leader in your organization about the philosophy related to case and disease management in your setting. Are there CMs or DMs in your organization? What about as part of the payer organization? See if you can interview or shadow a CM/DM for a half day.

3. Identify whether CPs are used in your organization and how they are developed and updated. What are the main information sources for the evidence used?

4. If you and your staff interact with CMs or DMs, consider inviting them to lunch or a staff meeting to discuss how you can work together better to enhance effective and efficient patient care.

REFERENCES

Baker, J. J., & Baker, R. W. (2004). *Health care finance: Basic tools for nonfinancial managers*. Sudbury, MA: Jones and Bartlett Publishers.

CMSA. (2005). Definition of case management. Retrieved May 13, 2005, from the CMSA website: http://www.cmsa.org/AboutUs/CMDefinition.aspx

Crosson, F. J., & Madvig, P. (2004). Does population management of chronic disease lead to lower costs of care? *Health Affairs, 23* (6), 76–78.

Cudney, A. E. (2002). Case management: A serious solution for serious issues. *Journal of Healthcare Management, 47* (3), 149–152.

DMAA. (2005). Definition of disease management. Retrieved May 13, 2005, from the DMAA website: http://www.dmaa.org/definition.html

Fireman, B., Bartlett, J., & Selby, J. (2004). Can disease management reduce healthcare costs by improving quality? *Health Affairs, 23* (6), 63–75.

Harrison, J. P., Nolin, J., & Suero, E. (2004). The effect of case management on U.S. hospitals. *Nursing Economics, 22* (2), 64–70.

Interqual Care Criteria. (2004). Description retrieved May 14, 2005, from the website: http://www.interqual.com

Milliman Care Guidelines. (2005). Description retrieved May 14, 2005, from the website: http://www.careguidelines.com

Powell, S. K. (2000). *Case management: A practical guide to success in managed care.* Philadelphia: Lippincott.

Radzwill, M. A. (2002). Integration of case and disease management: Why and how? *Disease Management & Health Outcomes, 10* (5), 277–289.

Ramsey, C., Ormsby, S., & Marsh, T. (2001). Performance improvement strategies can reduce costs. *Healthcare Financial Management* (Suppl.) 2–6.

CHAPTER 11

Improving Quality and Performance

Dori Taylor Sullivan

To use information and quality tools to continuously improve performance and create a culture of quality.

CHAPTER QUESTIONS

1. How and why were quality and performance improvement approaches introduced to health care organizations?
2. What are the major principles of quality and performance improvement?
3. What role do the management of information and information technology play in achieving the best results from improvement efforts?
4. How does the concept of evidence-based practice relate to quality improvement in general and in my area of responsibility?
5. Who are the significant accrediting and regulatory bodies influencing quality measurement in health care and what is their focus?

INTRODUCTION

In this chapter we discuss quality improvement as a business strategy along with ways to build a culture of quality. The clinical leader is the translator of organizational approaches to quality and plays a major role in identifying priorities for improvement, establishing and maintaining quality standards, participating in data collection activities for regulatory and accreditation purposes, and assuring that improvements are evaluated for safety, efficacy, and effectiveness. Perhaps most important the clinical leader is the key factor in creating a quality of culture, or a commitment to continuous improvement, in the microsystem. We should also note that measurement of quality, including client outcomes, can be a source of staff motivation and satisfaction as they document a job well done.

We give a brief overview of the evolution of performance improvement in health care followed by the major principles of quality and performance

159

improvement common to all the major approaches. Regardless of the specific quality improvement program that your organization has selected or developed, most of the principles will be applicable. For example, the commitment to data-driven decisions for improvement is universal. While the initial focus of performance improvement was on administrative processes, the practice rapidly spread to clinical systems and outcomes; so we discuss this as a special case of performance improvement.

We show how evidence-based practice is related to performance improvement and particularly the impact of the quality of available data to inform identification of best practices. Finally, we present a summary of what the major regulatory and accreditation agencies are requiring related to quality improvement, patient safety, and outcomes of care.

INTRODUCTION OF CONTINUOUS QUALITY IMPROVEMENT TO HEALTH CARE

Somewhere around 1980 the concept of quality assurance (QA) began to be popular in clinical settings in acute care hospitals. Early QA efforts were mostly a counting activity and, while carried out with the best intentions, tended to focus on aspects of care that were relatively easy to count rather than processes or outcomes of most interest to practitioners. These early QA activities received a lukewarm reception from most disciplines and were met with relative disdain from physicians. As is often noted by measurement experts, it seems that the easy things to measure are relatively unimportant, while those things that would really make a difference are difficult to measure and interpret. The fact that the focus of QA tended to be determined and imposed by a central authority was another strike against these early efforts. The result was general compliance with the mandates but little enthusiasm and limited use of the findings.

The Quality Movement and Its Translation Into Health Care

During the 1980s the work of Deming (1986) was noticed by health care leaders. Deming is considered the ultimate guru of total quality management (TQM), based on his work rebuilding the manufacturing businesses of war-torn Japan beginning around 1950. Deming promoted what he termed *constancy of purpose* and systematic analysis, with measurement of process steps in relation to capacity or outcomes. The TQM approach incorporated the view, as the name implies, that the entire organization must be committed to quality and improvement to achieve the best results—and to promote joy in work.

The staggering success of these improved Japanese businesses was first recognized by some industries in the United States, including manufacturing; slowly other sectors took note. Health care was a natural extension given the concerns about quality and cost of care that were beginning to accelerate. Soon after gaining popularity in health care, the quality improvement movement was translated into public and higher education. While some were quick to label quality improvement as a fad, it has flourished in health care and education and has become a business standard for success.

Besides Deming other experts quickly gained national prominence. New and existing consulting firms created or added quality and performance improvement consulting and education services to assist the many health care organizations eager to introduce these powerful methods. Juran (1988) and Joiner (1994) are two other widely recognized experts in quality improvement, both of whom lead international consulting firms devoted to quality management principles, culture, and techniques. Today the field is comprised of hundreds of trademarked approaches to quality, making it impossible to cover them all. We can, however, identify and discuss the most important principles of quality and performance improvement.

Language of Quality Improvement (QI)

First, a word about the "jargon" of quality improvement. Over time different terms became popular and then faded away as newer terms were embraced. The relatively early TQM was somewhat displaced by continuous quality improvement (CQI) and then by performance improvement (PI). Although there are distinctions made by the originators of these and other terms, for our purposes we will use *quality* and *performance improvement* to describe a comprehensive and formal system of principles, methods, and techniques to systematically measure and improve processes and outcomes. Also, how quality is defined differs somewhat among various approaches; however, virtually all definitions of quality include meeting or exceeding customer needs, decreasing variation, and minimizing or eliminating defects or errors from products or services.

Quality improvement may focus on enhancing existing processes or designing quality processes. When existing processes are believed to be incapable of yielding the desired results, redesign or reengineering of a process is undertaken. Hammer and Champy (1993, p. 22) explained reengineering as the "fundamental rethinking and radical redesign of processes to achieve dramatic improvements in critical, contemporary measures of performance, such as cost, quality, service, and speed." While there are clearly differences in improving versus redesigning a work process, we will use quality improvement (QI) to describe all such efforts.

Table 11.1 Principles of Quality Leadership

1. Customer focus
2. Obsession with quality
3. Recognizing the structure in work
4. Freedom through control
5. Unity of purpose
6. Looking for faults in systems
7. Teamwork
8. Continued education and training

(Scholtes, 1988, pp. 1–11)

Principles of Quality and Performance Improvement

Scholtes (1988, pp. 1–10) aptly notes that many elements of quality leadership have "appeared separately in fads that swept through business schools and organizations," such that many are unfamiliar with a comprehensive approach to performance improvement that has been termed "a new way of doing business." The principles shown in Table 11.1 and described below, as presented by Scholtes about the Joiner model, may be worded differently in various approaches but their meaning is the same.

Customer Focus

The customer is the center of quality efforts as an organization strives to meet or exceed customer goals and provide value. Quality approaches recognize external customers (the users of products or services) and internal customers (those within the organization that receive goods or services from other departments).

The translation of QI principles into health care requires that we think about the term *customer* a bit differently. In a strict business sense, customers are the ones who pay for the service or product they receive. The case in health care is more complex, since much of the cost of health care is borne by third parties including employers, insurance companies, and the government as opposed to clients themselves. And, frequently the goals and desires of clients are in conflict with those of the payers. Some have referred to the client as the ultimate customer, so as not to confuse where our primary obligation lies. That said, most health care organizations and their clinical managers typically try to identify and balance the needs of these major customers, which sometimes are conflicting.

A related principle in this customer focus is to measure, not assume or guess about, what customers need and want. This focus on data and information recurs in many of the quality principles.

Obsession with Quality

Everyone in an organization must be obsessed with quality! This principle may be best defined by the phrase *building a culture of quality* where the norm becomes the relentless pursuit of quality products and services through efficient and effective methods of execution. Building a culture of quality requires attention to staff education, clear communication of goals and expectations, provision of necessary resources, organizational systems that are efficient and effective, and alignment of performance and rewards systems.

Recognizing the Structure in Work

All work is comprised of processes that are structured not random. The structure and processes must be studied, measured, analyzed, and improved systematically to achieve the best results. Quality improvement includes specific tools and techniques to quantify and understand work, providing the data needed to create improvements.

To best understand the structure of work, management and staff must work together since each brings valuable information to the activity. We must appreciate that the people directly involved in the work have the best information about how that work is performed—and how it could be done better. In addition, the focus on work rather than individual performance engages staff in a positive way. This approach fundamentally changes the relationship between staff and management and fosters trust, respect, and empathy. You should recognize these as elements of transformation leadership.

Freedom Through Control

Quality improvement embraces the idea of quality control and reducing variation to produce regular desired results. Standardizing processes and ensuring that everyone uses those standards should make work processes more efficient and effective. The increase in productivity should allow for more freedom to develop new ideas for the business, enhance service to the customer, and improve skills in key areas. For example, in a clinical service area, if the scheduling procedure for clients is a refined and effective process, the scheduler or receptionist should not have to spend as much time on the telephone or negotiating with patients or providers, freeing up time for other important activities.

Unity of Purpose

Unity of purpose speaks to a clear and widely understood vision for the organization that unites or aligns all who work there. It is the vision that guides quality improvement efforts and provides criteria for decision making and problem solving when issues or opportunities arise. In a truly patient-centered health care organization, we would expect to see tangible efforts to promote comfort, safety, and timeliness. During a recent visit to an ambulatory surgery facility the following actions were noted. A sign in the reception area asked patients to come up to the desk if they had been waiting longer than 15 minutes to be called for registration. Upon changing into a hospital gown, patients were provided with two warmed bath blankets. While awaiting surgery, patients were asked if they wanted fresh warmed blankets, and blankets were also wrapped around a family member who was chilled. No one in that organization raised questions about the cost of providing this service, as patient satisfaction data clearly supported how much this amenity was valued, both for its physical comfort and communication of caring at a stressful time.

Looking for Faults in Systems

The QI philosophy and culture specifies aggressive continuous improvements of all work systems. The most important factor underlying this principle is accepting that systems rather than individual people are responsible for 80 to 85 percent of the results achieved (claims made by Deming and Juran, and supported by the Pareto principle or 80/20 rule). Loosely translated, the Pareto principle says that 80 percent of the poor results or troubles come from 20 percent of the problems. Or, as some managers like to say, 20 percent of their staff causes 80 percent of the problems!

Realistically, we cannot work on all systems at the same time so a way to identify priorities for improvement is essential. This is usually done through the collection of performance data on critical indicators across the organization (sometimes called a *dashboard report* or report card). In addition, departments create function-specific performance indicators that reflect improvement foci for specific areas. There needs to be some alignment or relationship between organizationwide goals and focus and those of the departments, since it is at the point of service within the departments that quality happens or not. An example of this alignment might be an organizational commitment to improving turnaround time. For radiology, this might mean the reading of reports. In the lab, the measure would be time until test results are available. In the rehabilitation department it might relate to readying special rooms or equipment between clients so there would be decreased waiting time and more appointments possible during a day.

Teamwork

There are few if any important work tasks that people do completely by themselves. Thus, we rely on others who play a part in supplying us with the products and services (including information) that we need to do our jobs well—or who need to work collaboratively with us to achieve the desired results. Teamwork differs from individuals or groups in that teams are defined having members who are committed to working toward a common goal or vision. The best team results are achieved when there is a diversity of ideas and relevant skills on the team that represent the important aspects of the work to be improved.

Continued Education and Training

An ongoing commitment to education and training across the organization is critical to keeping the culture of quality alive and thriving. There are always new techniques and ideas to be shared and enhanced skills for obtaining, managing, measuring, analyzing, and using information for improvement. Furthermore, education tends to make staff feel valued and important while enhancing their skills in a concrete way.

TOOLS AND TECHNIQUES FOR IMPROVING QUALITY AND PERFORMANCE

Improving quality and performance in any organization requires attention to three major areas: leadership, skills for gathering and using information related to work analysis, and the people factor. The Joiner triangle (Scholtes, 2003, p. xxi) in Figure 11.1 shows the relationship of these elements where quality leadership and the scientific approach represent the skills and tools for work analysis and improvement and "all one team" represents the people factor. Teamwork is at the heart of most QI efforts because teamwork reflects how work is typically accomplished and because more brainpower with different perspectives usually develops better solutions. We next present an overview of each of these areas so that you can consider the implications for your role as a clinical leader.

Figure 11.1   The Joiner Triangle

In Scholtes, P., Joiner, B., Streibel, B. (2003). The Team Handbook. 3rd Ed. Madison, WI, Oriel Inc., p. xxi.

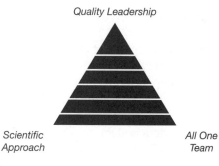

Quality Leadership

Scientific Approach

All One Team

Leadership for Quality

The role of leaders in an organization endeavoring to create a culture of quality and continuous improvement cannot be underestimated. Any serious initiative to create a quality organization must be sincerely embraced at the senior levels of the organization as well as by clinical leaders and be constantly reinforced through actions and reward structures, or what has been called *walking the talk*. Staff are experts at identifying inconsistencies in leader behavior, and they use any incongruence to decide whether to believe and invest in what is being proffered.

Scholtes (1988, pp. 1–14) identified six steps needed for quality leadership and a continuous improvement culture. Senior leadership must first commit to a rigorous education program for their team that addresses all three elements of the triangle. Second, they should define the organizational culture characteristics and values that they wish to develop that are consistent with continuous improvement. Third, senior leaders should develop a multiyear improvement strategy (two years is recommended) so that a pathway is clearly defined. The next step is a plan for educating the entire workforce, usually done in phases for logistical and cost reasons. This is a significant undertaking that when well done yields powerful results by introducing a new way of thinking about work improvement and relationships. Fifth, a formal network of support and guidance (often defined as access to quality facilitators with advanced knowledge of QI techniques) should be established and communicated. Finally, the specific improvement projects should be identified and initiated.

Similar processes at the microsystem level are needed to create a culture of quality and improvement at the unit level. Clinical leaders must encourage their staff to develop skills in QI and participate in defining and changing the unit culture as desired. A unit vision creates the context for a sequenced plan of improvement projects, identifying the resources within and outside of the unit needed to support these efforts.

Using the Scientific Method

In simple terms the scientific method can be used to test our assertions. More precisely, the scientific method is a set of orderly, systematic, controlled procedures for acquiring dependable, empirical—typically quantitative—information about a topic or question (Polit & Beck, 2004, p. 15). This method involves four steps after identifying a question or, in our case, a work process, to focus on: assessment and data collection, problem identification, interventions, and evaluation (Table 11.2).

Table 11.2   Steps in the Scientific Method

1. Assessment and data collection
2. Problem identification
3. Selection of interventions or solutions
4. Evaluation of results

Scientific Method Tools for QI

Some commonly used tools for data collection, analysis, and problem identification have evolved from the quality movement: traditional statistical control processes (mostly from manufacturing) and the discipline of management engineering. For our purposes, we describe only the most frequently used tools so that you can get a feel for this skill set. Our purpose is to introduce you to the tools. You can build your knowledge base by searching the Internet and/or working with your quality improvement department. Your charge is to determine the specific quality approach, methods, and tools used in your own organization so that your knowledge and skill development targets those specific areas.

Flowcharts. A flowchart is a diagram that uses standardized symbols to create a paper picture of steps and decisions that make up a work process. There are several variations of flowcharting but each serves the purpose of defining the detail and order of a process. Flowcharts may be developed as a team activity, or individuals may be assigned to create a flowchart based on their understanding of the work process. There are often conflicting opinions about process flowcharts, so one of the major purposes they serve is to develop a common view of an existing or proposed process, a first step in reducing variation.

Pie Charts and Pareto Charts. Most people are familiar with pie charts, which display the percentage of categories or responses using the wedges of a circle that look like slices of pie. The size of the wedge reflects the frequency or size of that category. Similarly, Pareto charts use the same information as a pie chart but depict the categories or responses in a bar graph that orders the named categories from highest to lowest in terms of frequency or impact. The purpose of the Pareto chart is to determine whether in each case the rule holds true, that is, 20 percent of the categories will explain 80 percent of the problems.

Cause and Effect (Fishbone) Diagrams. Fishbone diagrams are used to categorize and analyze possible problem causes related to a desired or problematic effect or outcome. The shape of the diagram resembles a fish with bones, thus the name. The fishbone diagram is a picture of lists with increasing amounts of detail as more "bones" are added to the descriptions of possible causative factors. As with flowcharts, cause and effect diagrams may be developed by the team or by individual/small group efforts and then compared.

Operational Definitions. Operational definitions specify a concept or element and how it will be measured. For example, a definition of good turnaround time for a pathology report could be more precisely stated as a typed, signed, final report delivered to the ordering physician within 72 hours of receipt of the specimen. Without precise definitions of effects or outcomes, it becomes difficult to measure the impact of various work process steps or issues.

Run Charts (Time Plots) and Control Charts. A run chart or time plot depicts a series of observations or measures of a work process over time. The purpose of seeing variations over time is to look for patterns that could lead to understanding causes of variation or diminished performance so that effective improvement strategies can be created. Recall that one of the first steps in QI is decreasing variation; the run chart shows the amount of variation over time. For example, the clinical manager of an emergency clinic wishes to see the number of patient visits by day of week so that he can develop a better staffing plan. A two-week run chart shows that visits are much higher on Thursdays, Fridays, and Saturdays. The next step might be to analyze time of day of visits for those days on a second run chart. A control chart is a run chart with boundaries for expected variation drawn into the display. The values for these boundaries are calculated from statistical control formulas that a quality expert could assist in determining. Variation within the boundaries is referred to as common cause or normal variation. Points of variation outside the boundaries are termed special cause and require further investigation.

Checksheets. Checksheets are forms developed to facilitate collection of observed data about a work process step or element. Checksheets should be as simple as possible with the goal of showing patterns or amounts easily. As an example, consider the case of a courier service that provides service to a freestanding nutrition center. The center might develop a checksheet to document whether the courier is on time and how many items he is delivering. This data could be used to decrease the service and reduce costs, or to investigate an improved method of accomplishing this activity.

Gap Analysis. A gap analysis is used to assess the nature and amount of difference between the current state and the desired state of designated characteristics or outcomes. The best gap analyses incorporate measurement data to support the description of the current state and definition of the desired future. For instance, if a goal is to have active participation in shared governance of a department, you could measure the number of staff participating on councils.

Root Cause Analysis. Root cause analysis is a formalized investigation and problem-solving approach focused on understanding the underlying causes of an event as opposed to focusing on symptoms of a problem. Root cause analysis seeks to determine what happened, how it happened, and why it happened, with the overall goal of making recommendations for prevention of future events. The four steps in root cause analysis are data collection, causal factor charting, identification of root causes, and generation of recommendations and implementation of changes (Rooney & Vanden Heuvel, 2004, p. 46). A root cause summary table may be used to summarize the findings and recommendations of the analysis.

The People Factor and Teams

Each of us has probably experienced an unproductive or uncomfortable group meeting, where differing opinions and dialogue did not result in a consensus or decision. Consensus may be defined as an idea or proposal that all team members can positively support, even though it may not be their personal first choice or preference. Achieving consensus is generally preferred to majority rules voting or an authoritarian decision because it promotes better solutions and improved team relationships as well as buy-in from members.

Team Communication and Decisions

Using structured communication and decision-making tools improves team functioning and outcomes. The tools and techniques described below are designed to promote efficient presentation of ideas and opinions after which agreements can be developed for how to proceed.

Brainstorming. Brainstorming is a technique that enables a group to generate and list many ideas within a short time period. It also promotes relatively equal participation, assuring that talkative members do not monopolize the discussion.

Participants contribute one item in order with no comments about the ideas allowed. People may pass if they have nothing to add during that round, and the session is stopped by time or lack of additional ideas. The group then clarifies their understanding of each idea and may combine similar items. The next steps are for the group to agree on criteria for evaluating these ideas or how to reduce the list to the best ideas to make it manageable.

Multivoting. Multivoting allots a certain number of votes to each participant that they use for their most preferred items from a brainstorming or other list. Multivoting reduces the list of ideas by retaining only those items with the higher number of votes. It is often used following a brainstorming session to focus the team on one or more items. After combining similar items, the remaining items are numbered. Each member is given a specified number of votes. Items with the lowest vote totals are eliminated and another multivoting session may be conducted; this process can be repeated as many times as needed.

Nominal Group Technique. This technique is a more formalized approach to determine priorities from a list generated by participants. It combines elements of brainstorming as participants write down their ideas independently in response to a question or topic. A master list of the ideas is compiled on a flipchart. Each participant is then asked to assign a rating or number of points to a specified number of the ideas presented. This technique is helpful for relatively new teams or controversial topics.

Affinity Diagrams. Creating an affinity diagram is an action strategy to develop categories or see how numerous elements might be related based on perceptions of a group. Each member is instructed to write down three to five responses to a question, writing each response on a separate sticky note. The individual notes are then posted on a large wall by all participants. Participants are instructed to group the sticky notes together as best makes sense to them without speaking to others. Each individual can move the sticky notes into whatever configuration he or she prefers, but the next person can come along and undo it. After a period of time the group tends to arrive at a "good enough" solution. The clusters of notes depict a number of broad categories or themes that emerge. This activity can promote enhanced understanding of underlying causes of issues.

Lessons Learned for Promoting QI Team Effectiveness

In addition to the structured QI tools just discussed, consideration must be given to how to structure team activities for the best outcomes, acknowledging that individuals have needs and motivations that may detract from team effectiveness. As a culture of quality develops in a unit or organization, the norm is to question and improve everything and defensiveness decreases. However, to promote optimal team functioning and outcomes, attention must be given to establishing a clear charge, selecting the team members, and assigning roles. These recommendations apply whether the team is from your unit or comprised of several departments across the organization, so make the appropriate adjustments depending upon the type of team.

Team Charge

Most organizations create a formal mechanism for deciding upon improvement priorities relying on appropriate performance data and quality indicators. Once the decision is made that a cross-functional team (comprised of staff from multiple departments or areas) should be convened to address an improvement opportunity, a formal charge to the team is prepared. This charge should include the specific nature of the improvement opportunity and the desired outcomes, timelines, resources available, team members, and any other parameters or assumptions the team needs to accomplish its charge. A team charge is similar to a team charter, differing only in how much detail is fleshed out by the person or group creating the team. Teams often create a charter from a general charge. Table 13.2 in Chapter 13 gives an example of a team charter.

Selection of Members

The selection of team members is crucial to team success. Individuals who have "process owner" status, meaning that they have primary responsibility for this work, must be included both for their knowledge and to promote buy-in for recommended improvements. If you want to establish a team on your unit to improve the response time of the night shift and you have a night charge person, it is essential to have the charge person on the team. Staff who actually perform the work and are closest to the provision of services should also be team members. Those who supply information, products, or services (suppliers) as well as internal and possibly external customers should also be represented, either as team members or through invitations to join certain meetings. The size of a QI team varies among organizations and projects, but most experts seem to agree that between seven and nine is the best number for team effectiveness.

Team Roles

There are six basic roles in a QI team: team leader or chair, team member, recorder, timekeeper, facilitator or quality adviser, and executive champion. Depending on the size of the team, some of these roles may be combined or even rotated; whatever the plan, the team needs to ensure that all the functions are assigned and carried out.

Team Leader. The team leader is formally in charge of the team's efforts including meeting schedules and agendas, between-meeting assignments, maintenance of the formal team records, and communication with others regarding the team's work (unless this is specifically assigned to a team member for specific requests). The team leader role may be performed by co-chairs if desired. The team leader works closely with the facilitator for guidance and feedback on team performance and next steps. Whenever possible, the next meeting's agenda and between-meeting assignments should be reviewed and documented near the end of the meeting.

Team Member. Team members accept responsibility for sharing their ideas and information, preparing for meetings, completing between-meeting assignments, committing to continued learning, and contributing to overall team effectiveness.

Recorder. It is highly recommended that the team's work be captured on flipcharts or smart boards so that all members can see and assist with what is being recorded. In addition, this method of recording eliminates the need to spend time writing minutes after the meeting, as meeting documentation can be typed from the recording sheets. Any reports or charts prepared may also be attached and distributed to foster the team's work progress. The recorder function may be assigned to a specific team member or, more often, it is rotated among members.

Timekeeper. As the name suggests, this team role is responsible for helping the team manage its time. Agendas should include suggested time allocations for each agenda item and/or the team should discuss how to best use the available time at each meeting. The timekeeper notifies the team when the allocated time has elapsed at which point the team can decide to stop the discussion or agree to continue for an amount of time.

Facilitator. The facilitator or quality adviser may be from the quality or education department or one of your colleagues who has received in-depth quality training. The facilitator has three main responsibilities. First and foremost, the facilitator works with the team leader to plan out the team's work and consider which QI tools or methods might be most helpful at different stages of the project. Second, the facilitator attends team meetings to observe and make recommendations to the team about their level of effectiveness and recommendations for enhancement. Many facilitators take five minutes at the end of each meeting to elicit members' perceptions of what went well and facilitated work versus what could be done better for the next time. Third, the facilitator is an expert in QI and provides formal or just-in-time training as needed to foster team progress.

Champion. Each QI team should have a senior leader appointed as the executive champion of the team's project. For unit teams, you as the clinical leader would be identified as the champion. Frequently, the team leader and the facilitator encounter issues or barriers that require assistance or advice from senior administration. And while the champion does not attend all team meetings, that person does establish regular communication and this provides information to show that the team is on track to meet the improvement goals. Table 11.3 provides a summary of QI tools and techniques, and Table 11.4 lists the team decision methods.

Table 11.3   Summary of QI Tools and Techniques

QI Tools	QI Techniques
Flowchart Pie chart/Pareto chart Cause and effect (Fishbone) diagram Operational definitions Run and control charts Checksheets Root cause analysis	Brainstorming Multivoting Nominal group technique Affinity diagrams Structured discussion

Table 11.4   Summary of QI Team Concepts

Team charge (opportunity, outcomes, timelines, resources, assumptions) Selection of members Size of team Team roles (leader, member, recorder, timekeeper, facilitator, executive champion) Ground rules

Ground Rules

Ground rules (or rules of engagement) evolve from team discussions about how members wish to behave with one another to promote member satisfaction and team success. Ground rules often include expectations related to prompt attendance, participation, interruptions (pagers and phones), decision making, conversational courtesies (such as no interrupting when others are speaking), and confidentiality agreements when appropriate. Once ground rules are established through consensus it is easier to hold members accountable for compliance.

WHAT MAKES QUALITY IMPROVEMENT SUCCESSFUL?

The traditionalist QI approaches developed by Deming, Juran, and Joiner, among others, remain the method of choice in numerous health care organizations. Others have opted to follow two newer models: General Electric's (GE) Six Sigma and Work Out® (GE, n.d.) and Studer Group's Pillars of Excellence (Studer Group, n.d.). The Six Sigma and Pillars of Excellence approaches have been adopted by growing numbers of health care organizations. These approaches while evolutionary in terms of QI retain the core principles presented earlier in this chapter.

Many QI approaches have led to spectacular organizational successes. The major factors in this success may be summarized into three themes. First is the commitment of leadership to the fundamental principles of quality, improvement, measurement, empowerment, and involvement. Leaders must visibly, powerfully, and continuously talk and walk the talk! Second, a clear and consistent model for QI should be selected and refined for use in an organization; this would also be used at the unit level. As you have seen, the QI field is cluttered with jargon and people become easily frustrated if the language changes all the time. Staff want to master QI skills and that is more difficult to do without a clear model, terms, and processes. Third, there must be an investment in building a quality infrastructure to provide the resources, human and material, required for QI success. As a clinical leader, you need to assure that your staff teams have sufficient resources and direction for success. You or members of your staff may also be asked to develop additional QI skills to support efforts throughout the organization.

Benchmarking is a term denoting the use of information from other organizations to use as a comparison or benchmark in evaluating an organization's performance. Benchmarking may be a relatively informal, collegial process or, more often, an extensive and detailed project. The utility of benchmarking data is enhanced when there are common operational definitions for key data elements and metrics for reporting. It also works better when the organizations, or at least the specific area or work process being benchmarked, share important characteristics.

Recently the emphasis in benchmarking has been on best or better practices. For example, if a hospital is trying to reduce length of stay for patients having total knee replacements, they should access information from a hospital having the lowest lengths of stay and excellent quality outcomes. This comparison yields two helpful things. It provides a reality-based sense of the possible in the current environment, and it allows for learning about how the length of stay reduction is achieved.

Many health care organizations belong to proprietary benchmarking service companies or groups and can regularly access performance data in areas of interest such as patient satisfaction. These comparisons may also facilitate the identification of organizational or departmental improvement priorities if there is a major difference in efficiency and/or effectiveness of the care or services under study.

Benchmarking is discussed in more detail in the section on accrediting and regulatory agencies' quality initiatives. We now turn our attention to the special case of clinical improvement and the related concept of evidence-based practice.

CLINICAL-PROCESS IMPROVEMENT AND EVIDENCE-BASED PRACTICE

The successes in administrative and support processes using QI skills led to transferring this approach to clinical processes and outcomes. While QI was largely driven by administrators at the beginning, physician leaders and other clinicians recognized the opportunities that a structured approach to improvement provided. Further, given the long tradition of a research-based approach to care, a renewed interest in using research evidence to guide care decisions and protocols developed. The term *evidence-based medicine* or *practice* was coined and reflects this renewed emphasis by medicine, nursing, and other health disciplines. We also note how advances in information technology have accelerated and supported clinical improvement and evidence-based practice.

Clinical-Process Improvement

Clinical-process redesign or improvement means "the effective design of the continuum of care to satisfy customers, improve patient outcomes, maximize efficiencies, and improve the organizational climate" (Strongwater & Pelote, 1996, p. ix). The specific outcomes of general interest specified by these authors include clinical outcomes, functional outcomes (physical, social, and quality of life), patient satisfaction, organizational climate (staff satisfaction and readiness to change), along with cost and utilization indicators.

As individual health care organizations identified clinical-process improvement as a major strategic goal, entities that support hospitals and other agencies developed clinical-improvement programs and resources to assist their constituencies. For example VHA, Inc., a national membership organization for community hospital systems, and the University Healthsystems Consortium (UHC), a member organization for academic medical center hospitals and systems, each created divisions for clinical improvement. VHA, Inc. and UHC added physicians, nurses, and other quality experts to their staffs to provide consultation and other resources to support their members' efforts. The development of comparative databases for benchmarking and creating peer relationships for learning and improvement blossomed during the 1990s, and entire conferences were regularly held to advance this area.

At about the same time, the Agency for Healthcare Research and Quality (AHRQ) came into being and began assimilating research to issue practice guidelines with the expectation of improving patient outcomes. The stated mission of AHRQ is to improve the quality, safety, efficiency, and effectiveness of health care for all Americans (AHRQ, n.d.). The AHRQ develops consensus around evidence-based best practices for priority health care concerns like pain, incontinence, and others. This brings us to evidence-based practice.

Evidence-Based Practice

Evidence-based practice (EBP) is the integration of best research evidence with clinical expertise and patient values to deliver optimal care (Sackett, Straus, Richardson, Rosenberg, & Haynes, 2000). Best research means clinically relevant, patient-centered research studies. Clinical expertise refers to the role of clinical skills and experience as well as unique patient presentations. The inclusion of patient values reflects the need to individualize care to meet individual preferences, needs, and concerns to best serve that patient. These authors further assert that to carry out EBP there must be sufficient research published on the specific topic of interest, the health practitioner has skills in accessing and critically analyzing research, and last, that the practice allows for implementing changes based on the evidence. Table 11.5 summarizes a five-step process for EBP.

The evaluation of evidence is often done using a system for grading or leveling the quality of the evidence according to accepted research standards. There are several systems for grading evidence with one example being a three-grade system that indicates:

- Level I or A—a multisite randomized clinical trial or several single-site randomized studies
- Level II or B—a quasi-experimental study
- Level III or C—a correlational or descriptive study

Table 11.5   Summary of EBP and the Five-Step Process

Evidence-based practice (EBP) is the integration of best research evidence with clinical expertise and patient values to optimize clinical outcomes and quality of life.

(Sackett, Straus, Richardson, Rosenberg, & Haynes, 2000, p. 1)

1. Formulate a question arising from patient clinical problems based on current knowledge and practice.
2. Search for and access relevant evidence or research.
3. Evaluate the evidence using established criteria for scientific merit.
4. Choose interventions or changes in practice, justifying the selection with the most valid evidence for the patient population it will be applied to.
5. Implement the change(s) and evaluate the results.

While EBP in health care is not totally new, the emphasis and widespread commitment to its use, facilitated by exploding and more readily available evidence, continues to grow and has become the standard of care. Another factor contributing to EBP is the time pressure experienced by most health care providers. Instead of having to go to a library, clinicians can use their PDAs or a computer with Internet access to quickly locate current research data and critical reviews on a particular topic. There are also evidence-based clinical guidelines available for purchase to guide practice in the field.

Recognizing that patient outcomes result from the efforts of numerous disciplines, the most effective EBP models combine the interventions of the involved disciplines for various patient conditions, although each discipline retains responsibility for assessing its own professional practice. For further information about current evidence-based improvement initiatives, refer to the websites for the Institute for Healthcare Improvement (www.ihi.org) and ZYNX (www.zynx.com) for examples.

Despite its popularity, some barriers to EBP have been identified, most commonly accessibility of research findings, anticipated benefits of using research, organizational support to use research, and support from others (Retsas, 2000). Health care organizations need to find ways to foster the culture of quality and support systems to make EBP a way of life to provide the best and most cost-effective care. Clinical leaders will be expected to use research knowledge and skills to promote safe, high-quality care. If you have not already done so, consider taking a formal or continuing education course to enhance your competence in this area.

Managing Information and Information Technology

The evolution of computerization and information technology (IT) in health care is a complex and interesting topic. For our purposes, we comment on the critical role of IT and some of the issues and decisions that will critically affect our ability to improve quality and enhance efficiency using IT advances. We expect that all readers have some experience with IT systems in their organizations whether it be for managing staffing or supplies, scheduling visits or procedures, tracking records, entering medical orders, or using electronic medical records.

One of the major issues in health care is the jigsaw puzzle approach to computerization in most health care organizations. For a variety of reasons, different departments or functions were automated at different times, after which more comprehensive software systems became available. Decisions related to interfacing abilities (getting the systems to talk to one another and share information) versus extinction of the original system in favor of wider benefits are quite common. Comprehensive software systems can now be purchased for many health care setting needs related to client medical records, tracking, services, payments, and outcomes; financial matters; staff and patient scheduling; and many others.

Automation tends to improve information access, communication, and documentation; decreases redundancy of data entry; facilitates the use of data for research and QI; and promotes easier compliance with regulatory requirements. Initial and ongoing costs of these systems along with information security can be significant challenges. Another challenge is called data integrity or verifying that the data in the system is accurately coded, entered, and available. While many health care organizations are making progress in implementing a fully automated medical record, most are still working at this process.

Leapfrog Group is a conglomerate of non–health care Fortune 500 company leaders committed to modernizing the current health care system (Milstein, 2000). This increasingly influential group has identified three evidence-based initiatives they believe will dramatically improve outcomes: (1) computerized physician order entry (CPOE), (2) evidence-based hospital referrals (EHR), and (3) intensive care unit physician staffing (IPS) (Hudon, 2003, p. 233). We discuss the first two, since they directly relate to subsequent content.

Implementation of a CPOE system addresses several components of medical errors related to medications, namely the legibility of orders, completeness of information, and the ability to use a clinical decision support system (CDSS) to cross-check for dangerous drug interactions or contraindications. Although evidence clearly supports improved quality and financial outcomes related to CPOE, the initial expenses are substantial. These statements could apply to many software systems available to health care agencies. Another factor is that most would agree that computerization often does not save professional time but does improve the quality and availability of data.

The EHR recommendation supports that consumers should have access to quality and outcome data for specific conditions and procedures so that they can make informed choices regarding where to seek care. We address this in more detail in the sections on regulatory and accrediting quality initiatives.

Clinical leaders will need to be involved in the implementation of systems that include their areas or serve their areas specifically. And it is generally recommended that representative clinical leaders and the staff on the frontline participate in the selection of software systems to provide the end-user perspective. Thus, enhancing knowledge of information technology systems and capabilities will lead to better use of information for evidence-based practice, quality, financial, and other purposes.

ACCREDITATION AND REGULATORY FOCUS ON QUALITY

The major accreditation and regulatory entities in health care have taken significant steps to promote quality and safety in the delivery of health care. Although many of the efforts focused on hospitals, they noted that other settings would likely have similar issues. Recommendations for assessing other settings (like nursing homes, ambulatory care, and home care) to identify differences and effective solutions were frequently encouraged. In this chapter we review some of the major changes and recent requirements that focus on improving the quality of care and patient safety with attention to cost effectiveness and service utilization, changes that have significant impact on clinical leaders in most settings.

JCAHO Performance Improvement and Safety Standards

The Joint Commission on the Accreditation of Health Care Organizations (JCAHO) provides voluntary accreditation services to hospitals, home-care agencies, ambulatory care, long-term care, behavioral health, laboratories, and office-based surgery, among others. The JCAHO should be credited for an early effort to require contemporary QI activities of their accredited facilities. As early as 1987, JCAHO's Agenda for Change called for demonstration of systematic QI efforts including "closing the loop" by evaluating the impact of improvement strategies. At the same time JCAHO began development of performance measures that evolved into the ORYX initiative, a requirement for benchmarking clinical outcomes of selected conditions.

Since 1999 JCAHO has met with stakeholder groups to develop a set of hospital core measures. Three initial major diagnoses were selected for testing after extensive pilot testing, feedback from pilot hospitals and information derived from the Centers for Medicate and Medicaid (CMS) of the United States Department of Health and Human Services (HHS). The three diagnoses are: acute myocardial infarction (AMI—9 measures), heart failure (HF—4 measures), and community-acquired pneumonia (CAP—5 measures). A fourth area, pregnancy and related conditions (PR), was added later as was the measure for surgical infection prevention (SIP). Additional measures are under development with the stated intent to stay consistent with CMS goals and initiatives.

Two other JCAHO requirements deserve mention in the context of quality and safety. JCAHO calls for a patient safety plan that reflects a comprehensive approach for reporting, analyzing, and preventing medical errors through a variety of actions. Specific attention is given to sentinel events, defined as "an unexpected occurrence involving death or serious physical or psychological injury, or the risk thereof" (www.jcipatientsafety.org). In an assessment of 2,966 hospital sentinel events reported between 1995 and 2004, JCAHO listed the top five root causes of sentinel events from all categories as communication, orientation and training, patient assessment, staffing, and availability of information.

For our purposes, and because of the role hospitals play in the current system, we have used the JCAHO accreditation of hospitals as an exemplar to illustrate how quality and safety requirements have evolved. As a clinical leader, you should become knowledgeable of the JCAHO or other accreditation agency standards for your areas, many of which have headed in similar directions. The next section summarizes reports from the Institute of Medicine (IOM) and highlights the information that drove some of these changes.

IOM Reports

Three reports among the many issued by the IOM of the National Academies fueled the focus on measuring and reporting quality and safety in health care. Each of these reports is briefly presented with the major recommendations.

The first of the three reports, *To Err Is Human* (IOM, 2000), drew major headlines with its finding that as many as 98,000 deaths each year in the United States were due to medical errors. This number surpasses the number of deaths from motor vehicle accidents, breast cancer, and AIDS. It was also reported that the cost of one category of these errors, preventable adverse drug reactions, was about 2 billion dollars. The goal of the report was to break what was called the "cycle of inaction" and improve the quality and safety of the delivery of health care in the United States. A four-tiered set of recommendations was made including:

- A national focus to create leadership, resources, tools, and protocols to increase the knowledge base on health care safety.
- Identification and learning from errors with mandatory reporting of events.
- Raising standards and expectations for improving safety among oversight organizations, purchasers of care, and professional groups.
- Creation of safer systems in health care organizations leading to safe practice at the level where care is delivered, the ultimate goal of all the recommendations.

The next pivotal IOM report, *Crossing the Quality Chasm* (IOM, 2001), called for fundamental changes to the health care system to increase the benefits of care while decreasing harm. It acknowledged that the current system does not make the best use of resources due to the impact of errors and overuse. The report also stated that the system is plagued by outmoded systems of work and called for public and private purchasers of care, health care organizations, clinicians, and patients to work together to redesign health care processes. Six aims for redesign of the health care system were established, indicating the new system should be safe, effective, patient-centered, timely, efficient, and equitable. The IOM also suggested that HHS take a role in identifying priority conditions and foster research and improvements in care delivery based on this knowledge. Finally, the report listed 10 principles to guide the redesign of the health care system:

1. Care should be based on continuous healing relationships.
2. Care should be customized based on patient needs and values.
3. Patients should have control with shared decision making.
4. There should be shared knowledge and a free flow of information.
5. Evidence-based decision making should be evident.
6. Safety should be designed in as a system priority.
7. There should be transparency to promote informed decision making.
8. The system should anticipate patient needs not just respond.
9. There should be a continued decrease in waste within the system.
10. There needs to be cooperation among clinicians.

Keeping Patients Safe

In its 2004 report *Keeping Patients Safe: Transforming the Work Environment of Nurses*, the IOM was asked by AHRQ to conduct a study with two aims: (1) identify key aspects of the work environment for nurses that were likely to have an impact on patient safety, and (2) recommend potential improvements in nurses' work conditions that would likely increase patient safety. This report emphasized the critical role that nurses play in patient safety and confirmed that the evidence supported that aspects of nurses' work environments were threats to patient safety. The IOM specifically noted the impact of reengineering or redesign in health care as detrimental by decreasing nurses' trust in administration and diminishing the voice of nurses in patient care at multiple levels. *Keeping Patients Safe* contains a wealth of detailed research evidence about many aspects of work environments and is worth reading in its entirety. Although the report targets nurses, many of the principles and recommendations can be applied to other health care providers. The report identified transformational leadership and evidence-based practice for management as two important concepts for improving work environments.

Specific recommendations were made in the areas of:

- Nurse staffing ratios and practices
- National data reporting of staffing
- Increased resources for knowledge and skill development from orientation through length of tenure
- Support for interdisciplinary activities that promote collaboration
- Limits on hours worked
- Design of work environments and care processes with a recommendation to first focus on medication administration and handwashing
- Creating an overall culture of safety within health care organizations

The later IOM reports built upon the work of the prior reports and had substantial impact on the health care system and professional communities. The imprint of the IOM report recommendations can be seen in later health initiatives.

CMS Initiatives

In November 2001 HHS and CMS announced the quality initiative designed to measure and report health care quality for consumer use with the support of Medicare's quality improvement organizations. The CMS launched the Hospital Quality Initiative in 2003, which aimed to define and standardize hospital data for collection, data transmission requirements, and performance measures. A 10-measure "starter set" focused on acute myocardial infarction (AMI), heart failure (HF), and pneumonia (PNE). Another 12 measures are under discussion under the auspices of the Hospital Quality Alliance (CMS, 2004).

Building on the Quality Initiative and work related to nursing home quality, pilot testing of improved measures for nursing home quality occurred in 2002 and 2003. It was reported that about 3 million elderly and disabled Americans received care in approximately 17,000 Medicare and Medicaid certified nursing homes in 2001. As of January 2004 the CMS Nursing Home Quality Initiative listed 14 quality measures on its Nursing Home Compare website for comparison in the areas of delirium, pain (acute and chronic), pressure sores, decline in activities of daily living, bedfast, worsening anxiety or depression, incontinence, indwelling catheters, mobility decline, physical restraints, urinary tract infections, and weight loss. New initiatives in the creation of staffing quality measures and background checks for employees are under development.

The CMS Home Health Quality Initiative was launched in 2003 to assess and report on quality measures for the significant number of individuals receiving home care services. About 3.5 million elderly and disabled Americans received care from nearly 7,000 Medicare certified home health agencies in 2001 (CMS, 2003). The home care quality indicators rely heavily on data provided from the Outcomes and Assessment Information Set (OASIS) introduced in the late 1990s to fulfill provisions of the Balanced Budget Act (BBA) of 1997 related to prospective payment for Medicare patients. The OASIS assessment purports to include core items of a comprehensive assessment for an adult home care patient and provide data for purposes of outcome-based quality improvement. The National Quality Foundation (NQF) is working with CMS on additional measures that are likely to include improvements related to ambulation, bathing, transferring, managing oral medications, pain interfering with activity, dyspnea, urinary incontinence, acute care hospitalization, discharge to community, and emergent care.

In the ambulatory care domain, CMS is again working with the NQF to endorse a set of standards, building on work initiated by the CMS and the American Medical Association's Physician Consortium for Performance Improvement, of the National Committee for Quality Assurance. The standards are expected to address asthma and respiratory illness, depression and behavioral health, bone conditions such as osteoporosis, arthritis, diabetes, heart disease, hypertension, prenatal care, and prevention/immunization/screening activities (CMS, n.d.).

Additional quality measures for other health care settings are in the JCAHO and CMS standards as well as in other accrediting and regulatory bodies' published information. Clinical leaders should access these other quality standards relevant to their areas. We have presented an array of current activities to underscore the wide and intensive efforts underway to measure and report quality, since it is a major responsibility of health care leaders.

Medicare Pay for Performance Initiatives

CMS is developing and implementing a set of pay for performance initiatives to support QI in the care of Medicare beneficiaries. CMS is focusing first on hospitals, physicians, and physician groups to be followed by home health and dialysis. As part of a demonstration project, incentive payments will be made to hospitals that demonstrate high quality based on data from 34 quality measures relating to five clinical conditions. A similar demonstration project began in selected physician practices across the country in spring 2005. More information about other pay for performance proposals can be accessed on the CMS website.

In summary, there is increasing evidence that the health care system is fragmented, unacceptably unsafe, and costly. The mounting evidence and public attention have led to unprecedented cooperation among major accrediting, regulatory, and professional groups to address this evolving crisis in health care. As you consider the information just presented, please reflect on the congruencies among the priority areas identified by major agencies like JCAHO, AHRQ, and CMS. Today evidence-based management and decision making are identifying clearer priorities for health care improvement. In addition, there is a comprehensive effort to include all settings where health care is delivered, especially important considering the shift of services outside of hospitals in recent years.

IMPLICATIONS FOR CLINICAL LEADERS

Clinical leaders are at the cutting edge (some might call it the bleeding edge!) in assimilating and acting on quality and performance standards for their areas driven by external forces (primarily accrediting and regulatory agencies) and internal mandates (health system corporate entities and organizationwide goals). Success in this area calls for balancing scientific or data-driven changes for improvement with the human side of the equation, recognizing that it takes time for people to embrace change. The creation of a culture of quality can enhance the staff's ability to positively improve care, control costs, and accelerate the pace of change that is needed.

As a clinical leader, you will need to hone your skills and commitment to mastering the skills of QI so that you can serve as a resource and role model for your staff. You will also be called upon to have an up-to-date knowledge of the current and expected quality measures that relate to areas you manage. The detailed planning for compliance with quality reporting depends heavily upon information management and technology, both systemwide applications and unit-based software systems.

While all these changes in QI and public reporting can feel a bit overwhelming, they are introducing a new era of excitement by refocusing health providers on our mission through outcomes-based QI and enhancing the care delivered to our clients. The systematic use of evidence to support or redefine how to best provide care is energizing and supports interdisciplinary collaboration. This focus on quality care and outcomes is assisting health care organizations to reinvent themselves and cut through the status quo system (or existing system) that no longer serves us or our patients well.

APPLICATION EXERCISES

In this chapter we expand the application exercises instead of using a scenario so that you can customize your activities to reflect your unique responsibilities. This will also give you a chance to practice your ability to apply transformational leadership, LIQ, and complexity theory to your practice.

1. What is the culture of your organization as it relates to QI?
2. Describe and name the overall approach to QI that is used in your organization. What is the nature of your participation in QI?
3. What are the most significant external quality standards or measures for your area(s) and from which accrediting or regulatory bodies are they derived?
4. Are there other quality measures for your area required by your own organization? If yes, what are they and why were they created?
5. What role does information technology play in your ability to efficiently and accurately access data to assess and report quality measures? Is this a strength or weakness for your area? For your organization?
6. Identify a current quality concern or improvement opportunity within your scope of responsibility and then consider the following questions:
   - Is there evidence to support considering a change?
   - How would the principles of transformational leadership assist you in moving this effort forward successfully?
7. What LIQ roles would you demonstrate in leading this project?
8. How might complexity theory tenets inform your planning and activities?

REFERENCES

AHRQ (Agency for Healthcare Research and Quality). (n.d.). *Mission statement*. Retrieved May 10, 2005, from AHRQ website: http://www.ahrq.gov

CMS. (2003, March 21). *Home health quality initiative overview.* Retrieved from the CMS website: http://www.cms.hhs.gov/quality/

CMS. (2004, January). *Nursing home quality initiative.* Retrieved from the CMS website: http://www.cms.hhs.gov/quality/

CMS (Centers for Medicare and Medicaid Services). (2004, November 22). *Building on the foundation: Hospital measures for public reporting,* CMS fact sheet. Retrieved from the CMS website: http://www.cms.hhs.gov/quality/

Deming, W. E. (1986). *Out of the crisis.* Cambridge, MA: MIT Center for Advanced Engineering Study.

GE (General Electric). (n.d.) *Six sigma.* Retrieved May 5, 2005 from the GE website: http://www.ge.com/sixsigma/keyelements.html

Hammer, M., & Champy, J. (1993). *Reengineering the corporation: A manifesto for business revolution.* New York: HarperCollins.

Hudon, S. (2003). Leapfrog standards: Implications for nursing practice. *Nursing Economics, 21* (5), 233–236.

IOM (Institute of Medicine). (2000). *To err is human: Building a safer health system.* Washington, DC: National Academy Press.

IOM. (2001). *Crossing the quality chasm: A new health system for the 21st century.* Washington, DC: National Academy Press.

IOM. (2004). *Keeping patients safe: Transforming the work environment of nurses.* Washington, DC: National Academy Press.

Joiner, B. L. (1994). *Fourth-generation management: The new business consciousness.* New York: McGraw-Hill.

Juran, J. M. (1988). *Juran on planning for quality.* New York: The Free Press.

Milstein, A. (2000). *Statement on behalf of the business roundtable.* Retrieved May 16, 2005, from http://www.brtable.org/document.cfm/372

Polit, D., & Beck, C. T. (2004). *Nursing research: Principles and methods (7th ed.)* Philadelphia: Williams & Wilkins.

Retsas, A. (2000). Barriers to using research evidence in nursing practice. *Journal of Advanced Nursing, 31* (3), 599–606.

Rooney, J. J., & Vanden Heuvel, L. N. (2004). Root cause analysis for beginners. *Quality Progress,* July, 45–53.

Sackett, D. L., Straus, S. E., Richardson, W. S., Rosenberg, W., & Haynes, R. B. (2000). *Evidence-based medicine: How to practice and teach EBM (2nd ed.).* Edinburgh: Churchill Livingstone.

Scholtes, P., Joiner, B., Streibel, B. (2003). The TEAM Handbook. 3rd Ed. Madison, WI: Oriel Inc.

Strongwater, S. L., & Pelote, V. (1996). *Clinical process redesign: A facilitator's guide.* Gaithersburg, MD: Aspen.

Studer Group (n.d.). Health care flywheel. Retrieved May 15, 2005 http://www.studergroup.com/$spindb.query.2flywheel.studview

CHAPTER 12

Human Resource Management Model

Anne M. Barker

To manage a talented diverse workforce in an environment that fosters staff satisfaction, growth, and achievement of clinical unit goals.

─────── **CHAPTER QUESTIONS** ───────

1. What are the eight major concepts in the human resource model and what are my responsibilities in each?
2. How do I use the model to work with others using transformational leadership and Leadership IQ as the guiding leadership strategies?
3. What are the organizational considerations that I have to keep in mind when using the model?

INTRODUCTION

Most of your work as a clinical leader involves working with other people to achieve your unit's goals. In this chapter, and the next one, we consider the role competency of leading and working with others. We do not particularly like the term "managing human resources," as it seems contradictory to the philosophy of transformational leadership and complexity science. However, after a long search for alternative wording, we are using the well-accepted terminology for this competency. We suggest you think about this competency as managing the structures, systems, resources and tools to optimize human capital, rather than as managing and controlling people. In this chapter we present a model to do this. The next chapter covers specific strategies to provide an environment where people can work together productively.

THE HUMAN RESOURCE MANAGEMENT MODEL

To optimize people assets, you need a systematic way to think through the activities that are involved in managing human resources. Many of the processes covered here you will be doing in collaboration with the Human Resource Department, which requires that you be familiar with and follow organizational rules and policies. The purpose of this section is not to discuss the mechanics of the processes in managing human resources, but rather to emphasize your role and responsibilities in carrying them out as a transformational leader.

We emphasize that as you engage in the activities presented here that these must be consistent with and support your unit vision. In Chapter 9 we suggested that the work environment for your unit should be one of the dimensions of the vision statement. For instance, most vision statements speak to providing an environment in which employees can thrive and be successful. Thus, when doing a work analysis, the first step of the model, your goal is to look at the delivery system and the people so that you can achieve this vision. Second, each step must also have as its ultimate goals how the activities will enhance relationships with your clients. This holds true for each of the steps in the model:

- Work analysis
- Staffing
- Selection including recruitment and interviewing
- Staff development, which includes orientation, competencies, reselection, and succession planning
- Evaluation—both informal and formal (performance appraisal)
- Staff retention
- Rewards including money and nonmonetary recognition
- Disciplinary actions and termination

Work Analysis

Conducting a work analysis means having the right people with the right skills in the right job at the right time to deliver quality, cost-effective care within budget (Murphy, 1996, p. 3). This involves determining future workforce requirements, assessing the current workforce, identifying the gaps between the future and current workforce, and developing strategies to close these gaps (Woodard, 2001, p. 36).

We encourage you to conduct a work analysis for your unit at this time as a baseline. If you have not yet developed a vision, then you should first start with a vision and then move to this analysis since you need to align the vision with the human resources needed to achieve the vision.

Once you have this baseline, you should review and revise the analysis annually when you prepare your budget for the upcoming year. Another important time to use the analysis is when you have a vacancy and are recruiting new staff for your clinical unit. This is an opportune time to think about the skills needed for your unit and to find the right person to fill the gap or adjust the skill mix by reconfiguring the number and types of positions to best reflect the work to be done.

The work analysis includes an analysis of many facets. First, the clinical manager should get a broad perspective by looking at:

- Organization mission, vision, and values
- Unit mission, vision, and values
- Future plans for the organization and your unit
- Customer needs and satisfaction
- Quality and performance data
- The external environment

Next, you need to consider the work to be done and the skills needed for the work. The best information about this comes from the staff that is doing the work. You can collect information both informally and formally. Informally, you can gather a lot of rich data by shadowing and talking with the staff as they are doing the work to find out what is and is not working well. Formally, by doing a written survey you can see trends and prioritize the changes that need to be made. Table 12.1 is a work analysis questionnaire that you can use to survey the staff.

Table 12.1   Work Analysis Questionnaire

1. List the three top activities in which you spend your time?
2. What are the roadblocks for you in getting your work done?
3. What wastes your time?
4. What is working well?
5. What is not working?
6. How much time do you spend daily on paperwork? How much duplicative paperwork do you do? Where can we streamline documentation? Is there anything you believe we could eliminate?
7. Do you have the appropriate and enough equipment to get your work done? If not, what are the top three priority areas for resolving equipment-related issues?

Other comments you would like to share:

With the data from this process you should conduct your own assessment and prepare a written report that:

- Lists the functions and work activities that occur on the unit. Think about what wasteful work may occur in your unit (see below).
- Lists the employees on the unit and their strengths, competencies, and skill/knowledge deficits. Assess the educational levels, experience, and skills of the staff to determine current and future needs.
- Considers both the present and future and whether there is enough, too many, or too few of any type of employee.
- Considers the competencies that are needed and whether the current staff have the competencies needed for today's work and for the future.
- Considers who should be doing what. Does the skill level required of the tasks match the expertise and education of the worker?
- Considers the complexity of each of the roles to determine if there is role focus or role overload.
- Assesses a different constellation of roles if suggested by the work analysis.

Work Analysis: Wasteful Work

There has been much interest in work analysis and wasted work in health care in recent years. This is due to several factors including the health care labor shortages that demand we utilize highly skilled and educated staff appropriately, delegating unskilled tasks and eliminating time wasters. Further, the concern regarding medical errors has required that health care leaders look at management systems to decrease errors and to have the skilled professionals in the right place at the right time.

A study of 71 hospitals conducted by the Murphy Leadership Institute (Murphy, 2003) found that, on the average, hospital employees spent 35 percent of their time on wasteful work that adds no value to organizational outcomes. This wasted time affected every discipline in the hospital including but not limited to nurses, pharmacists, managers, technicians, and housekeepers. The top 10 time wasters were:

- Duplication of paperwork. In a separate study Hicks (2001) found that every hour of patient care delivered in a health care organization generates 30 minutes to one hour of paperwork.
- Inefficient reporting from shift to shift and between departments.
- Interruptions by telephone calls.
- Finding equipment. In another study Gelinas and Bohen (2002) found that health care workers report that as much as 10 percent of their time is wasted on equipment-related issues such as slow computers and software systems that require more work than paper systems, broken

equipment, and not having enough essential equipment such as IV poles, blood-pressure cuffs, and wheelchairs.

- Unavailable and delayed medications.
- Long meetings.
- Searching for misplaced medical records.
- Unnecessary or redundant communications.
- Waiting for physicians.
- Waiting for something from another department.

Work Analysis: Matching Skill Levels

In a study of role design related to RN turnover, the VHA analyzed the job roles of 5,200 registered nurses in 137 acute care hospitals. They looked at skills and clustered them into two categories: clinical activities needing a low skill level and clinical activities needing a high skill level. Table 12.2

Table 12.2   Skill Level of Clinical Activities for Registered Nurses

Low Skill Level

- Feeding/assisting patients with meals
- Setting up equipment, an initial
- Assisting in patient transfers
- Distributing nourishment
- Bathing/skincare
- Toileting
- Changing linen
- Admitting/registration clerical activities
- Transferring/discharge clerical activities
- Collecting specimens

High Level Clinical Activities

- Assessing patients
- Serving as a preceptor
- Conducting case management activities
- Making professional judgment
- Supervising others
- Responding to codes
- Administering blood products
- Teaching procedures or treatment
- Developing discharge plans
- Consulting with physicians

Adapted from Gelinas, L., & Bohen, C. (2002). Designing work for optimal care promotes patient safety and staff satisfaction. *Clinical Systems Management, 4* (7), 13–15.

lists these skills. The interesting finding was that nurses who spent most of their time on low skill activities had the highest turnover, whereas nurses involved in the highest skill activities tended to stay in their employment area (Gelinas & Bohen, 2002). Although this is a study of nurses, we feel that this study also informs the other clinical disciplines and suggests that skill levels are an important consideration when doing a work analysis for any clinical discipline.

This study suggests that health care leaders must better utilize unlicensed assistive staff for doing the lower skill tasks. Unfortunately, there have been many issues regarding the increasing numbers of unlicensed staff including skilled staff who are unwilling and unable to delegate appropriately, conflict and unresolved feelings between the two groups, and the competencies of the unlicensed staff. However, it is simply essential that these issues be resolved through better recruitment, training, relationship building, and setting expectations since there will be a shortage of licensed skilled staff in many health care disciplines in the future.

Staffing

The next step in the model is to consider how you will determine staffing levels for your unit. The goal is to develop and implement plans to provide the level of care needed to ensure a safe environment for your clinical unit. We introduce you to the larger considerations for developing staffing plans and patterns so that you will have an understanding of the rationale behind the various approaches to staffing. Your organization most likely will have forms, formulas, and practices specific to its needs.

In our discussion we primarily use acute care situations because they are the most complex, requiring 24 hours/7 day per week coverage. The basic principles remain the same for all other settings and can be easily modified for them if you grasp the concepts at this more complex level.

In determining the staffing needs of a clinical unit, the first step is to calculate the *staffing pattern*, which is defined as the number of persons in each job classification that should be on duty per shift per day. Table 12.3 is an example. To calculate a staffing pattern, you need data about three areas: patient care requirements, unit characteristics, and characteristics of the staff.

Patient care requirements are determined in one of three ways. The first and most popular is to determine the *staffing hours per patient day*. This mathematical formula has been used in nursing for decades but can be used for any clinical discipline. However, its usefulness is seriously questioned as it

Table 12.3   Sample Staffing Pattern for an Acute Care Unit

	S	M	T	W	TH	F	S
Days							
Clinical Manager	0	1	1	1	1	1	0
Shift Manager	1	1	1	1	1	1	1
RN	4	4	4	4	4	4	4
PCA	2	2	2	2	2	2	2
RT	1	1	1	1	1	1	1
PT	0.5	1	1	1	1	1	0.5
Secretary	1	1	1	1	1	1	1
Housekeeper	0.5	1	1	1	1	1	0.5
Evenings							
Shift Manager	1	1	1	1	1	1	1
RN	4	4	4	4	4	4	4
PCA	2	2	2	2	2	2	2
RT	1	1	1	1	1	1	1
PT	0.5	0.5	0.5	0.5	0.5	0.5	0.5
Secretary	1	1	1	1	1	1	1
Housekeeper	0.5	0.5	0.5	0.5	0.5	0.5	0.5
Nights							
Shift Manager	1	1	1	1	1	1	1
RN	3	3	3	3	3	3	3
PCA	1	1	1	1	1	1	1
RT	0.5	0.5	0.5	0.5	0.5	0.5	0.5
PT	0	0	0	0	0	0	0
Secretary	0.5	0.5	0.5	0.5	0.5	0.5	0.5
Housekeeper	0	0	0	0	0	0	0

does not account for acuity, the other activities of the unit, appropriate skill mix, or delivery system.

$$\frac{\text{All personnel / 24 hrs} \times \text{No. of hrs worked}}{\text{Number of patients}}$$

The primary advantage of this method is that it is easy to calculate. The major disadvantages are that it does not discriminate for acuity, and it is based on the actual care provided versus the required care needed.

The second method is the use of patient classification systems. These were used extensively in the 1980s to determine patient care requirements on a daily basis. Many nursing units still determine patient categories daily but more likely they are used for long-term budget planning rather than for daily staffing. This does vary from setting to setting however. Patient classification systems categorize patients into groups based on their acuity and the required hours of care they need. There are many different systems used from home grown to proprietary, computerized to hand calculated, and descriptive and subjective to objective checklists.

The third way to determine patient care requirements is to consider historical data/consensus. In this method you determine what the staffing has been for the past year and how it should be adjusted. Using this method includes integration of the opinion and expertise and even intuition of the clinical manager. Most likely to some degree all three of the above methods are used in most settings.

The next step in looking at staffing is to consider the characteristics of the unit. Table 12.4 lists unit characteristics to be considered in different settings. In outpatient and community settings, the visit type (usually described in relation to time and complexity) is the standard metric for staffing considerations. The more visit types available, the more complex the staffing plan projection becomes due to the variability.

Next you need to consider the characteristics of the staff. This includes

- Staff expertise and level of experience and competency.
- Education and preparation of the licensed and unlicensed staff.
- Tenure on the unit.
- Degree of involvement in quality initiatives, research, inter-displinary and collaborative activities regarding clients.
- The number and competencies of clinical and non-clinical support staff that must be supervised.
- Skill mix or licensed and unlicensed staff.
- Type of care delivery system. For instance in nursing it may be functional, team, primary, primary team, or patient-focused care.

Table 12.4   Unit Characteristics for Staffing

Inpatient Settings

- Number of beds
- Average daily census
- Occupancy rate
- Type of unit
- Census fluctuation
- Unit architecture and geography
- Availability of technology

Home Care Settings

- Number of patients
- Number of visits per patient
- Average daily census
- Census fluctuations
- Average length of visit
- Average visits per employee
- Travel time
- Shifts and weekend visits
- On call
- Availability of technology

Clinic Settings

- Number of patients
- Number of visits per patient
- Average length of visit
- Number of exam/treatment rooms
- Hours of operation
- Availability of technology
- Clinic architecture and geography

One of the major problems in developing staffing patterns is that an underlying assumption is that patient care requirements are stable because we are working with averages. Since this is seldom the case, agency or temporary staff and float staff are a way to address this problem, along with extending hours and using overtime. Of course, each of these alternatives has some negative consequences that must be managed.

The next step, developing a *staffing plan*, is a bridge between the staffing pattern and the budget. It is using mathematical formulas to determine how many people of what job classification to hire to deliver on the staffing pattern.

Because employees generally work five days per week, have time off, and use sick leave, you have to hire more people than what your pattern says you need.

At its simplest level, if you need to have one person on duty on the day shift seven days per week, you need to hire 1.4 people to cover days off. This could be one full-time staff and a .4 part-time person or it could be any combination of individuals working part time to total 1.4 full time equivalent (FTE). For example, for the shift manager in the sample staffing pattern in Table 12.3 one individual is assigned to this position every day. Thus, for this clinical unit, 1.4 FTE would need to be hired to cover this position on the day shift. The same is true for evenings and nights.

The next step is to figure out how many other days off need to be covered (nonproductive time off), including sick leave, vacation leave, holidays, educational days, and others. This varies from institution to institution based on polices and average use for the institution regarding leave. Generally to do this calculation you would get the institution's averages from the Human Resource Department.

Selection

The next aspect of our model is selection. One of the eight roles of the leader using Leadership IQ as the framework is the selector role. For our purposes in this section we discuss the initial hiring and selection of new staff based on the principles of Leadership IQ. LIQ suggests that the purpose of selection is to have a good fit between the potential employee's values, goals, and abilities and the goals and needs of the organization and its customers. It is more important to choose the person with the right attitudes and values; training for skills can be offered if needed.

Before hiring into a position, it is crucial that the clinical leaders start with a work analysis and examine how the position should be configured to maximize its focus on priority elements. Once this analysis has occurred, it is easier to specify the ideal candidate.

Recruitment

Although you may not have the final decision about recruitment activities for your organization, an understanding of these is important. The following types of recruitment activities are widely used:

- Advertising in local newspapers and on the Internet.
- Providing financial incentives such as sign-on bonuses, relocation bonuses, employee referral bonuses, seasonal bonuses, off-shift bonuses.

- Offering enhanced benefits packages that might include loan forgiveness and flexible scheduling.
- Attendance at career days at colleges and job fairs.
- Holding in-house open houses.

As the clinical leader of your unit, you should participate in as many recruitment activities as possible. For example, when advertisements are posted for your clinical unit, you should give input so that the advertisement matches the needs you determined in your work analysis.

Interviewing

Interviewing skills are the key competency to develop in order to select the right person for your unit and the job. Two major types of interviews are popular. Both have the same purpose, which is to determine if the person has the attitudes and values that will enhance your unit. Although skills are important, they are secondary. You can always train and educate for skills, but you can never change someone's value system or personality.

We strongly advise you to include the staff in the interviewing and selection process. The Advisory Board Company (2001) suggests that this is not only a good strategy for selection but also for retention. There are three reasons for this. First, the staff may be able to get better and more honest information from candidates than you can as the manager. Second, applicants will have the opportunity to question the staff to assure that the position is a good fit for them. Ultimately, this will decrease turnover on your unit. And, third, when the staff is involved in the selection, they will more readily "buy into" the person, giving the person support to be successful as it reflects on their decision-making skills. Should there be a problem, some of the negativity is deflected from you, since the team is responsible.

Before an interview look at the person's application and resume. During the interview you do not need to ask about the information that is already on the resume, but instead clarify anything that is unclear and then move onto questions that will elicit information about the person's attitudes or personality. Be prepared with a list of questions that you have developed specific to your unit and its needs.

One type of interview is called a *behavioral interview*. In this type of interview the applicant is asked to cite specific examples demonstrating use of particular behaviors or skills. The applicant is asked to describe in detail specific events, projects, and/or experiences and how he or she dealt with the situation. By doing a search, you will find that there are many Web sites with long lists of behavioral interview questions that you can modify for your purposes. Table 12.5 has some sample questions to get you started, but it is not meant to

Table 12.5   Sample Behavioral Interview Questions

- Tell me about a goal that you have set in the past, what you did to accomplish it, what roadblocks you faced, and how you overcame them.
- Describe an experience you have had with a patient or co-worker that was a conflict and how you solved the problem.
- Tell me about your experiences in supervising patient care associates from diverse backgrounds. How did you relate to them and work with them?
- Tell me about an experience in which you felt that you delegated well to a patient care associate.
- Give me an example of when you were faced with a difficult decision in your job and how you dealt with it.
- How do you organize your work?
- Think about a problem patient and/or family that you had to deal with and tell me how you have handled it.
- Tell me about a time that you went beyond the normal job expectations in order for you to get your work done.
- What did you do in your last jobs to contribute toward the team?
- What three words would you use to describe yourself?
- What motivates you the most?

be a comprehensive list or even an appropriate one for your needs. In fact, the questions you ask should be specific to your unit's needs and be derived from the work analysis of the position and what you are looking for in the applicant. Thus, interview questions that you use for one position may not be the same interview questions that you use when filling a different position.

The second type of interview is called a *work history review* (see Table 12.6). By reviewing the applicant's work history, you can uncover the person's talents and abilities, core values, and career motivators. This information is much more useful than a classic resume review and discussion because it is intensely personal and revealing while creating a beginning relationship with a potential employee. The process steps or roadmap (see Table 12.6) provides a consistent and efficient guide for you to determine the likelihood of the applicant being able to make positive contributions to your work unit.

A work history review elicits patterns of an individual's positions, and it is usually easy to identify themes from the activities they enjoyed most and sought versus those they judged to be less satisfying or negative. The themes themselves are not inherently positive or negative, rather it is the fit between those patterns and the needs of the current position that should be assessed. For example, if you are starting a new program, it would be wonderful to have a new staff member who is high on self-directedness and initiative. In a medical staff or patient billing office, attention to detail and deriving satisfaction

Table 12.6 Work History Review

Instructions: Repeat each of these questions for each position change that the applicant has made. Include decisions to go to school, to work part time, or to not work at all.
- What was your first job?
  - Can be nonpaying
  - Be sure to get the title and major responsibilities of each subsequent job
- Why did you decide to do this?
- What did you like best about the job?
- What did you like least?
- How long did you perform that role?
- What did you do next?

from order and consistency might be more valued. For more information about interpreting this type of interview, refer to the classic work by Schein (1985) on career anchors.

When you interview, it is important to keep in mind the legal questions you and your staff can and cannot ask. You should get guidance from your Human Resource Department. In general, you cannot ask questions that would cause a person to believe she is being discriminated against for family status, race, religion, residence, sex, or disability. Some legal questions can be asked in these areas, but they must be asked of all applicants. For instance, you can ask a person his address, but you cannot ask who else lives there. Since the nuances of this are detailed and may vary, our best advice is for you to seek support from Human Resources. If you have your staff involved in interviewing, you must also make them aware of this issue and train those staff you have selected to do interviewing.

When you interview applicants, you should have a form to document the interview. Each applicant should be asked the same set of questions, and notes should be taken in a systematic format. When doing a group interview, one person can be assigned to take the notes. This person should be used as consistently as possible when interviewing candidates for the same position. This will assure consistency and allow you to compare each candidate based on criteria.

Staff Development

Most staff development activities focus on the development and verification of the clinical competencies of the staff. This activity is mandated by JCAHO standards. Further, the recent public concerns regarding medical errors and patient safety dictate organizations assure that health care professionals practice competently.

Competencies can be defined as the skills and knowledge required by the practitioner or employee in a given position to care for clients appropriately and safely. In general, when initially developing the competencies for your clinical unit you will need to consider high volume procedures, high risk procedures, and areas in which problems arise.

Next you will develop a competency checklist, usually in collaboration with your Education Department, which includes a brief description of the competency, a place for the employee to perform a self-assessment and have input, a definition of select learning activities in which the employee can engage to develop the competency, and a place for verifying and documenting that the employee has successfully demonstrated the competency. Your goal is to have a manageable list of competencies that reflect the core procedures and equipment used on your unit.

Once a person demonstrates initial competency there is no need to continually reverify these. Rusche, Besuner, Partusch, and Berning (2001) suggest that ongoing verifications should occur by exception. In other words there is no need to reverify either high-risk or high-volume procedures unless a problem has been identified by quality improvement activities, your own observations, or by concerns raised by the staff or patients. Rather, the focus of ongoing competency development is on less frequently used procedures in which staff needs to keep up their skills and do not have the opportunity to do this through daily practice. Further, another area of ongoing competency development, quite obviously, is when new procedures or equipment are introduced into the clinical unit. In summary, the focus of ongoing staff development should be on staff learning and growth and on problem areas.

Orientation

Staff development begins with the orientation process for new employees. Most organizations have a formal orientation program that involves orientation first to the organization, then to the department, and last, but most importantly, to the clinical unit. Depending on how educational services are organized, you may have responsibility for some or all of the unit orientation process. Your role is to assure that a new employee participates in orientation, completes the competency verification process, is socialized into your clinical unit, and ultimately becomes a fully contributing member of your unit.

Orientees can be evaluated by observation, by simulations, by returned demonstration, and so forth. Your role is to assure that this is done appropriately and timely, either by the centralized staff development department, the unit preceptor, or yourself. Evaluation should be ongoing throughout the formal orientation period. The orientation should conclude with a formal written evaluation. If there are problems or a need for employee growth, a plan for action should be developed by the employee and agreed to by all parties.

Performance Evaluation

As we discussed in Chapter 3, many clinical managers feel uncomfortable with their responsibilities for performance evaluation. Judging the work of others, especially recognizing our own imperfections and weaknesses, can be challenging and difficult. We would like to see you focus on this role and responsibility as a positive versus negative process by understanding that the overall goal of the performance appraisal (LIQ evaluator role) is to enhance individual performance. Performance evaluations are an opportunity to:

- Reward performance verbally and monetarily.
- Motivate employees by setting high expectations by developing goals that promote professional growth.
- Inform the employee of organizational and unit vision and goals.
- Define the role of the employee and how she fits into the overall success of the organization.
- Establish responsibilities and expectations for performance.
- Establish goals for future professional development.

The evaluator role in LIQ uses five principles to support effective evaluation. The first is to establish a clear purpose for evaluation, namely for the customer. Second, recognize that each individual is responsible for his behavior choices, including the choice to change or improve. Third, involve everyone in appropriate evaluation activities to promote a shared organizational value related to evaluation. The fourth principle calls for the necessary guidance or development for positive involvement. And, fifth, maintain focus on service—the fact that workleaders serve those who serve the customer (Murphy, 1996, pp. 116–120).

Performance evaluations need to be honest and thoughtful. Murphy (1996, p. 120) found that high-performing workleaders were more willing to recognize high performance and had wider variations of ratings among staff, reflecting their commitment to honest communication to foster improvement. These high but not unrealistic expectations foster a positive work environment that in turn attracts other high performers.

Process of Performance Evaluation

The process of performance evaluation is an ongoing one with three distinct phases. The first is planning, which involves meeting with the employee at the beginning of the evaluation period to communicate expectations and to determine mutual goals and objectives. Significant time should be given to this activity since it is more important to plan for the future by setting expectations than to evaluate the past. The primary purpose of looking at past performance is to improve future performance. The goals for the employee should be:

- Specific and relevant to the position
- Measurable
- Realistic and attainable
- Focus on results not activities
- Contribute to the overall clinical unit's goals and objectives

The second phase of the process is ongoing coaching, review, feedback, and discussions with the employee. These can be short informal interactions with an employee as well as more formal meetings. This approach is also an effective retention strategy.

The third phase of the performance appraisal process is the annual meeting with the employee at the end of the evaluation period. This process should be a partnership of the clinical manager and the employee with the employee conducting a written self-appraisal to provide input into the final performance evaluation.

Performance Evaluation Form

In this section we will not describe the different forms or tools used for performance appraisal in organizations. It is unlikely that you will be designing such a tool, but rather most likely you will be using one required by the organization in which you work. However, some characteristics of the tool that are important include:

- Customer focused
- Relevant
- Specific
- Clear
- Allow for two-way exchange
- Allow for performance improvement/development plans through goal setting
- Include both a self-assessment of the individual and the assessment of the clinical manager

Although you may not be able to modify the form you are required to use, you can independently adopt these principles in your performance evaluation process. For instance, you should include client outcomes and satisfaction in both the evaluation and goals. You can ask the staff for a written self-assessment whether or not the organization requires this. Likewise, you can develop goals for the employee independent of the organizations's form if need be.

Retention

The leadership strategies suggested and discussed throughout this book are, in their whole, retention strategies that provide a culture of trust, commitment, and meaning for staff. No one strategy stands on its own but rather is the gestalt of the clinical unit that you create. In summary, staff needs to have control over their practice, have a voice related to client care and care delivery, feel that their work has a direct impact on client outcomes, enjoy positive work relationships among the team, and be able to grow and learn.

In this section we discuss several activities related to retention not covered in other parts of the book. Like the other leadership strategies, these processes on their own and in isolation will not result in improved retention. It is your leadership, the overall climate of the unit, and relationships among the staff that will result in low turnover and high morale.

Retaining the New Hire

Since the highest turnover in most organizations is new hires, they need to be supported in socialization to the clinical unit. There are two strategies you can use to decrease this turnover. The first is to involve the staff in interviewing and selecting new employees. The second is having a preceptor program. When done correctly, these programs have been cited as the best strategy for orienting new hires, supporting them in the transition, building their commitment to the organization, and decreasing turnover of this group.

Characteristics of effective preceptor programs are as follows:

- They should be formal programs with appropriate resources devoted to them at both the organizational and unit level.
- Preceptors should be hand selected for their attitude and commitment to the unit, not just their technical skills.
- Preceptors should be appropriately trained.
- Preceptors should be recognized informally and formally using programs and processes available to you in your organization.
- Preceptors should be given the time to do the job with a reduced patient assignment.
- Preceptees should not be counted in the unit staffing for some agreed upon time period. Obviously, newly graduated practitioners will need a longer time than seasoned practitioners.

- There should be a formal system to document skill acquisition and competencies.
- There should be systems to support the new employee in socialization, role adjustment, and role transition as needed.

We recognize that you may or may not have a centralized preceptor program for the organization. If you do, you should work with the education specialist in implementing it on your unit and be a supporter of the program by following its processes. In this way you can also have input into how it works, what needs to be changed, what is and is not working so that it is useful to you. No matter what centralized systems are in place, you should not abandon your responsibilities to the new employees; plan to schedule frequent meetings with them.

If you do not have a formal, centralized preceptor program you can still incorporate the major concepts listed above on your unit by appointing and training unit preceptors, finding ways to reward them within your organizational polices and procedures, having written orientation documents for your unit and skills checklists, and adjusting the daily assignments for the preceptor and the new hire.

Retention Diagnosis

A second strategy specific to improving retention is to diagnose turnover risks by doing a retention assessment (Advisory Board, 2001). Using a spreadsheet or table, list all employees and what their risk of leaving is. Make plans for interventions for each at-risk employee. Table 12.7 is a sample worksheet that gives some of the major reasons for staff turnover.

Other Strategies

Throughout this book other strategies are discussed that directly impact on retention. We do not want to repeat these in any great detail but want you to understand that these activities are also important according to the Advisory Board Company (2001):

- Assessing systems and unit operations and implementing changes to remove obstacles and dissatisfiers.
- Setting up systems for open and continuous communication and connections.
- Team development activities both social and work related.
- Relationship building among the team with particular emphasis on physicians.
- Maintaining adequate staffing levels and appropriate workload.

Table 12.7   Sample Retention Assessment Worksheet

Name of Employee	Retention Risk	Plan of Action
Charlotte	Nearing retirement and discussing the possibility of leaving in the next six months.	Meet with Charlotte and suggest part time or occasional status. Suggest a move within the organization to a less physically demanding environment.
Andrew	One of the more senior staff; does not seem to be looking or thinking about moving. Likes new program development and opportunity to do that in another setting would be interesting to him.	Meet with Andrew to discuss his goals and needs. Involve him in a new unit project.
Catherine	Has announced her retirement in one year.	Meet with Catherine to discuss opportunities for part time or occasional status after retiring.
Bobby	New employee. At risk as a new employee. New position is quite different from previous one. Needs further growth and development.	Meet with Bobby to discuss his status and interest in staying. Develop plans for growth and development. Assign him a mentor.
Kate	Completing her education at the next level. At risk to leave for new opportunity.	Meet with Kate to discuss her plans. Design a new position that will meet her needs and those of the unit.

Rewards and Recognition

There are two times when managers tend to use rewards and recognition the most. First is when someone is exceeding expectations—a star performer. The other time is giving recognition to someone who has made an effort to improve performance. But between these two groups lay the majority of employees who meet expectations but who are often missed by the formal and informal recognition systems.

Behavior reinforcement theory (Skinner, 1969) informs us that if you want a person to repeat a behavior you should recognize it and praise it. Likewise, if you want a person not to repeat a behavior, you should punish it or ignore it. Unfortunately, what often happens is that we inadvertently ignore a behavior that we wish to be repeated. Thus, the clinical leader should be recognizing all employees for those behaviors that meet your expectations and that you wish to have repeated.

Human beings crave recognition. Most of us wear an invisible sign on our chests that reads, "Recognize me and appreciate me!" And the most powerful way for managers to do this costs nothing—words of praise are all it takes. Here are some guidelines for doing this:

- Provide feedback often. Consciously set aside time every day to find people doing the work you want to reinforce and recognize this work.
- Provide feedback as soon as you observe the behavior you wish to reinforce.
- Know what each employee considers appropriate feedback and tailor your feedback. Some people prefer to be recognized privately while others enjoy public recognition. However, public feedback has the advantage of reinforcing your standards and expectations.
- Provide recognition that is proportionate to the behavior, sincerely given.
- Think small. Find the person doing something right, not perfectly (Grote, 1995, pp. 48–50).

Although words are one, if not the most, effective mechanism for recognizing and rewarding staff, there are other ways to do this. The list of ways to recognize people is inexhaustible and you probably use many different techniques to recognize people—from buying a cup of coffee to giving free coupons and certificates as well as the formal system of merit review and special awards. What we encourage you to do is make sure that these processes are given fairly and equitably to promote satisfaction and high morale not resentment.

To conclude this section, we would like to review an important theory regarding staff motivation. Herzberg's (1966) classic theory of job satisfaction and dissatisfaction still informs how we recognize and reward people in organizations today. Herzberg states that job satisfaction and job dissatisfaction are not direct opposites but are separate related entities. Herzberg identified factors that caused employees to be dissatisfied, which he called hygiene factors, including such things as company policy, administration, salary, supervision, interpersonal relationships, and working conditions. On the other hand, factors that cause people to be satisfied with their work, called motivation factors, include elements that people need to grow and develop such as achievement, recognition for achievement, advancement, the work itself, and responsibility. What is important is that if you eliminate a factor that causes dissatisfaction, the person will be less dissatisfied, but will not necessarily feel increased satisfaction. This is an especially important concept to understand when using money as a means to increase satisfaction; it does not work. If you increase salaries, people will become less dissatisfied with their salary, but this does not mean they will become satisfied with their work unless the motivation factors are positive. Thus, having competitive salaries sends the message that "we value you" and can decrease dissatisfaction to assure that people won't leave the job for a higher salary elsewhere. However, as the clinical leader you must attend to many more issues than money alone to keep the staff satisfied.

Discipline and Terminations

This aspect of human resource management is most likely one of the most distasteful and difficult tasks of your role. Most likely you have a formal system of progressive discipline designed by your organization that starts with informal discussion, which then moves to a formal verbal warning to written warning(s) to suspension, ending in termination. In a unionized environment the contract will outline the steps to be taken and the timelines. Whether you are in a union environment or not, you should seek advice and support from the Human Resource Department through each step of the formal process.

These systems were designed to build a case for terminating employees to assure third parties that people have been made aware of their deficiencies and given appropriate time and training to correct them. Thus you must follow the steps closely.

Grote (1995, pp. 14–18) suggests that this system generally promotes the following scenario. Progressive discipline sets up an adversarial relationship between the employee and the manager that breeds anger, apathy, resentment, and frustration. Because of this, managers often do not take action until it is clear that they must and have no alternatives. At this point they view the likelihood of the employee changing her behavior as hopeless. Thus, when the manager finally takes action it is to build a case for termination versus assisting the employee to change and be successful. The manager generally wants to move quickly through the process since termination now seems inevitable; he or she becomes frustrated by the process which can take significant time.

Types of Behavioral Problems

Grote (1995, p. 57) proposes that all problem behaviors fall into one of three mutually exclusive categories. If you use these three categories, it will help you to determine your coaching approach and how long you will wait to move forward to use the formal system. For example, you may be more tolerant of someone seriously trying to correct an attendance problem than of an employee who has stolen equipment. Grote's categories are as follows:

- Attendance. The organization expectation is that employees report on time for work, stay the full shift, and come to work as scheduled.
- Performance. Performance expectations include quantity, quality, cost, and time. For health care, employees need to carry an assignment concomitant with their background and education (quantity), and clients should experience positive outcomes from their relationship with the employee without complaints and with satisfaction (quality). Employees need to do this in a cost-effective way without waste and complete their work in a timely way so that daily work is completed.
- Conduct. These expectations can include such things as theft, drug diversion, accepting gifts, and not following the organization's code of conduct.

It is important to understand that you cannot intervene to change a person's attitude. That is because attitude is internal and basically cannot be changed. But attitude drives behaviors and relationships with others. Thus you should identify and focus on the behavioral problem that a negative attitude produces.

Coaching Problem Employees

The focus of this discussion is to have you reframe your thinking about the disciplinary process from looking at it as building a case for termination to working with and coaching problem employees based on a value of helping the employee to change and to meet organizational expectations. When you do this, you can decrease your anxiety about the process and thus intervene earlier and not ignore problems until it is too late. To do this, you should:

- Focus on correcting problems not punishing them. Your job is to coach employees by making performance expectations clear and helping them to understand how their performance affects the unit.
- Confront a problem employee in ways that maintain and enhance self-esteem.

- Influence the person to change behavior by having him accept responsibility to meet performance expectations.
- If necessary, provide training and remove obstacles that prevent high performance.
- Provide feedback when more improvement is needed and give positive reinforcement when the employee's behavior meets standards.
- Document coaching sessions. This may be notes for your own files and future reference, which are not for the employee. If you believe you need to give the employee a written confirmation of the coaching session and the plan of action, you can do this, however, just like the verbal interactions, you need to keep the tone of such a letter supportive and helpful. Before giving an employee something in writing, it would be wise to review this with your boss and the Human Resource Department to assure you are in compliance with policies, government regulations, and union contracts.

You have the discretion to decide when informal coaching is not working and when you have to go to a formal disciplinary system. But even then you should view the steps as a way for the employee to be rehabilitated versus being terminated. In this way as you work through the process you can still focus on having the person accept responsibility for his behavior and maintain self-esteem thus keeping the process less dissatisfying for you and less adversarial.

SCENARIO

John Bell is the clinical nurse manager of a 20-bed medical unit that is being expanded to 30 beds. He has been given a budget to hire six new RNs. With the opportunity to hire new staff, John decided to complete a work analysis before deciding on the staffing mix, job requirements, and beginning recruitment. First, he reviewed the organization mission, vision, and values as well as those for the clinical unit. Next, he looked at the current customer satisfaction results, projected future customer needs, and reviewed quality and performance data. He went to a meeting at the local hospital association about the current projected labor supply and demand and the development of new roles for nurses. In summary, he determined the following:

- The population in the community is not only growing but aging and is expected to have an increase in chronic illnesses.
- There is a current and projected shortage of RNs in the community.
- Clients will be in need of health care in the home as well as on his unit.

- Current patients are satisfied with the quality of the care related to technical interventions and caring attitudes, but are dissatisfied with communications related to education and preparation for discharge.
- Quality data demonstrates a high urinary infection rate and a moderate rate of medication errors.

Armed with this information he was now ready to talk with the staff. He first talked informally with as many staff as he could to ask them how they envisioned the new growth and how it could occur consistent with the unit vision "to provide world-class care to their patient population." He asked the staff to consider how this new growth could provide an opportunity to do things better and in new ways. In these conversations he included the information he had discovered in his initial assessment.

He then conducted a written survey asking the questions listed in Table 12.1 of this book. He found that nurses spent the majority of their time:

- Administering medications and monitoring IVs
- Monitoring patients' vital signs
- Dealing with hygiene and nutrition
- Documenting care
- Admitting/registration clerical activities
- Transferring/discharge clerical activities

Next John appointed a team to make recommendations as how to best spend the new money for the unit. The team made the following recommendations:

- Hire a part-time clerk whose primary responsibilities would be admitting, transferring, and discharging activities. The clerk would work in the late morning and early afternoon during the time of heaviest activities.
- Hire three patient care assistants, one for each shift, to assume responsibilities for the lower level skill activities.
- Hire an RN to serve as educational specialist/special project coordinator for the unit charged with orientation of new hires, ongoing education assisting the RNs to learn how to delegate, coordinating quality improvement activities, collaborating with the staff to improve patient education and discharge planning.
- Hire 2.5 RNs with the remaining money.

SCENARIO ANALYSIS

As a transformational leader John assured that the vision of the unit and the organization would guide the work analysis and ultimate decisions. By involving the staff from the initial assessment to making recommendations, he developed trust by providing an opportunity for mutual decision making and goal setting.

Using complexity science, he understood his role to be that of "sense maker." He compiled a lot of information initially so that he could help the staff understand the internal and external environments in which they practiced and to prepare them for the future. For instance, because of the nursing shortage hiring six RNs may be unrealistic. By hiring clerical and nonlicensed staff, the work of the unit can be accomplished differently.

Fulfilling the selector role in LIQ means he will need to set up an interviewing system to select the right people for the unit. Once again, we see that the effective leader uses many roles to accomplish the work, in LIQ principles this is the "synergistic kick."

APPLICATION EXERCISES

1. Conduct a work analysis of your unit to attain baseline data. Ask the staff to complete the questions in Table 12.1. From their answers, set some specific strategies for your unit.

2. Review the staffing plan and pattern for your unit in light of the work analysis.

3. Assess the orientation program for your unit.

4. Conduct a retention assessment analysis using the template in Table 12.7.

REFERENCES

Gelinas, L., & Bohen, C. (2002). Designing work for optimal care promotes patient safety and staff satisfaction. *Clinical Systems Management, 4* (7), 13–15.

Grote, D. (1995). *Discipline without punishment.* New York: American Management Association.

Herzberg, F. (1966). *Work and the nature of man.* New York: World Publishing Company.

Hicks, G. (2001, May 7). AHA study: Each hour of care can equal one hour of paperwork. *AHA News.*

Murphy, E. C. (1996). *Leadership IQ.* New York: John Wiley & Sons.

Murphy, M. (2003). *Research brief: Eliminating wasteful work in hospital improves margin, quality, and culture.* Retrieved February 28, 2005, from Murphy Leadership Institute website: www.murphyleadershipinstitute.com/pdf/murphy-wastefulwork.pdf

Rusche, J. D., Besuner, P., Partusch, S. K., & Berning, P. A. (2001). Competency program development across a merged health care network. *Journal for Nurses and Staff Development, 17* (5), 234–240.

Schein, E. H. (1985). *Career anchors: Discovering your real values.* San Diego: University Associates.

Skinner, B. F. (1969). *Contingencies of reinforcement: A theoretical analysis.* Englewood Cliffs, NJ: Prentice-Hall.

The Advisory Board Company (2001). *Becoming a chief retention officer: An implementation handbook for nurse managers.* Washington, DC: Author.

Woodard, J. W. (2001). Three factors of successful work force planning. *The Journal of Government Financial Management, 50* (3), 36–38.

CHAPTER 13

Human Resource Management Strategies

Anne M. Barker

To manage a talented diverse workforce in an environment that fosters staff satisfaction, growth, and achievement of clinical unit goals

---

CHAPTER QUESTIONS

1. What is conflict?
2. What strategies are available to help manage conflict between myself and others in the organization and conflict among the staff in my clinical unit?
3. Why is it important to understand intergenerational and cultural diversity in my clinical unit?
4. What are the stages of team development and what is my role in helping the team to learn, grow, and work together?
5. What should I consider when communicating with others?

INTRODUCTION

In this chapter we look at some of the most common strategies for leading and working with people. These include conflict management, working with a diverse workforce, team building, and communication. We focus on the concepts and principles that make each of these strategies distinct. However, all of them are done within the context of transformational leadership, Leadership IQ, and complexity. Further, these strategies overlap. For instance, you can use the strategies for managing conflict when working with diversity differences or team disagreements.

CONFLICT MANAGEMENT

Conflict can be simply defined as a disagreement between two or more people who differ in attitudes, values, beliefs, or needs. Further, the parties involved in the conflict are interdependent, meaning that the conflict cannot be resolved without mutual effort (Masters & Albright, 2002, p. 14). Conflicts can range from minor disagreements to union strikes.

It is a well-accepted fact that conflict will and does exist when two or more people work together. Most organizational experts agree that conflict is inevitable and necessary to allow differences of opinion and approaches to emerge. If managed successfully, resolution of the conflict can lead to better ideas and problem solutions. This means that conflict and differences must be handled correctly. Conflicts that are not managed appropriately will have many negative consequences including decreasing morale and self-esteem, polarizing people and groups, and making the work environment unpleasant and dissatisfying.

Although you may expect the ultimate goal of managing a conflict is to eliminate it, in fact, your goal for resolving a personal conflict or interceding in the conflict between others might be one or more of the following:

- Preventing escalation of the conflict
- Solving the real problem that underlies the conflict and clarifying important problems and issues
- Depersonalizing the disagreement
- Building relationships by involving people in resolving issues important to them and communicating openly and authentically
- Releasing negative emotions and relieving anxiety
- Achieving the unit's goals (Masters & Albright, 2002, pp. 72–73).

Analyzing the Sources of Conflict

We want to emphasize that the approach you use to manage a specific conflict should be reflective and thoughtful. In other words you should be proactive versus reactive in resolving a conflict. The first step is to analyze the specific source of the conflict so that you can take preventative steps. If you do not engage in this analysis and identify the source of the conflict, you may choose incorrect strategies or involve the wrong people in resolving the disagreement.

Organizational conflicts can arise from a variety of sources. Masters and Albright (2002) provide a useful framework for diagnosing sources of workplace conflict. They categorized these sources into environmental, individual, organizational, and workplace sources. *Environmental sources* include economic, legal/regulatory, cultural and generational demographics, and political/social sources. *Individual sources* of conflict arise from the personality, values, and beliefs of the members of the organization. *Organizational sources* of conflict arise from the need of the organization to be profitable and productive, the governance and leadership of the organization, its structure, and its ownership. *Workplace sources* arise from the work itself, technology, the workforce, and working conditions.

Determining Conflict Strategies

Conflicts can arise from interactions at all levels in the organization and from others external to the organization. Conflict can occur among individuals and between units or departments. As the clinical leader you will need skills both in managing conflict when you personally have a conflict with others as well as skills in mediating conflicts among the staff and in developing the staff to handle conflicts on their own.

Most conflict resolution scholars and practitioners agree on five basic strategies for resolving conflict:

- Accommodation
- Avoidance
- Competition
- Compromise
- Collaboration (Masters & Albright, 2002)

Each of these strategies can be used, but each has its strengths and weaknesses. However, for whatever strategy you choose, you need to do this in a proactive, reflective way, putting aside feelings of anger or hostility. The timing of conflict resolution is important as you want to approach it as objectively and unemotionally as you can. Thus, at times you might need to step away from the situation and people involved to gain a perspective on the issue.

We briefly describe the first four strategies and suggest when each can be used. When choosing which strategy to use, you must honestly assess the situation and desired outcome and the relationship with the other person or people. You also should be aware of your organizational culture and what strategies are valued. Choosing the wrong strategy will result in negative consequences. The last strategy, collaboration, is the most important and should be used in most situations. For this reason, greater emphasis is given to this strategy.

Accommodation

With this strategy, one of the individuals in the conflict accommodates or concedes to the other's position for the purposes of settling the disagreement.

Accommodation is a strategy reserved for situations in which you place a low importance on the issue or outcome and want to preserve and nurture relations of those involved.

Avoidance

This strategy is one, unfortunately, that is often overused. One or more of the parties in the conflict ignores or denies the conflict. This strategy can be used when you place a low importance on both the issue and the relationship. However, you must be careful not to avoid a conflict because it is unpleasant. Avoidance can often breed resentment and build long-term hostility.

Competition

When competition is the strategy, one person selfishly persists until he "wins" at the expense of others. This obviously can breed resentment and hard feelings that can fester for a long time. Its use is limited to those situations in which you place a low importance on the relationship with the other party and a high importance on the outcome. Choosing this strategy does not mean that you need to be hostile, angry, or divisive when using it.

Compromise

In this situation, both parties settle for less than their desired outcome. Compromising can be used when you place a medium importance on both the task and the relationship.

Collaboration

This is generally the preferred method for conflict resolution. Since it takes time, energy, and the willingness and skills to work with one another, it may not be the first option that people choose. With collaboration as the strategy, the goal is to find a win-win solution to the disagreement that is satisfying to everyone involved. It is both outcome and relationship focused. Because the goal is for everyone to be satisfied with the outcome, collaboration inherently means being willing to talk through issues, to be open minded, and willing to change one's mind or preferences. Without this willingness it is generally impossible to find a win-win.

Masters and Albright (2002, p. 79) suggest that collaboration should be used when the following criteria are met. For most conflicts that you face as a clinical leader these conditions exist:

- Relationships are important and interdependent.
- Mutual interests exist.
- Outcomes are important.
- Maintaining the team is important.

- The nature of the work is integrated.
- Cultural, professional, and occupational differences exist.
- Potential for the conflict escalating is high.

Steps for Collaboration. These steps have been adopted and modified from the work of Masters and Albright (2002). They can be utilized in three ways: to resolve a conflict between yourself and another person(s); to facilitate a conflict resolution among your staff; and to advise the staff how to resolve their own conflicts when appropriate for them to do so.

Resolving conflicts using collaboration means that the involved people must meet face to face. In the steps that follow individuals meet at least twice, but more if the disagreement is complex.

Step 1. Diagnose, analyze, and prepare. First, you should step back and take time to think about the sources and causes of the conflict. Reflect on what you believe to be the values, beliefs, and needs of the people involved. If you are part of the conflict, think about your own values, beliefs, and needs. During this phase you should gather information that you need and prepare your strategies for meeting with the others involved in the conflict.

Step 2. Set up a meeting to discuss the situation. In this first meeting you should sit back and listen, looking for the feelings, emotions, and thinking processes behind what is being said. Your goal is to understand everyone else's perceptions since everyone perceives the world and issues differently. If you are involved in the conflict, you also need to present your own feelings and opinions by focusing on facts, your value system, and the vision. You should avoid placing blame on individuals and keep the discussion depersonalized. Unless the conflict is minor, the meeting should be adjourned so that everyone can reflect on what they learned at the meeting.

Step 3. Capture the situation. Again, conflict resolution requires thinking and analyzing. You now need to analyze what you heard at the meeting looking for where the conflicts in values and beliefs exist, identifying the core issues, and identifying the facts. You also need to analyze where people's values and beliefs are similar, as this will provide the basis for resolving the conflict. You should encourage everyone else to do the same so that when you move to the next step everyone better understands one other.

Step 4. Explore, analyze, and plan. You are now ready to explore options, assess and analyze the options, and propose a plan. Depending on the complexity of the conflict this may happen in one meeting or many. The goal is to have everyone speak, be heard, and to reach consensus.

Step 5. Build relationships. Once the conflict is resolved, efforts still should be made to build relationships, to explore what was learned from the situation, and what did not go well.

DIVERSITY

In this section we focus on cultural and intergenerational diversity. The goal of managing diversity is more than avoiding discrimination, increasing the representation of minorities, and "celebrating differences." The goal is to use the varied talents and perspectives that individuals with different cultural and generational experiences bring to the workplace. This can result not only in increased organizational effectiveness, but also in improved morale.

Cultural Diversity

Cultural diversity refers to the many racial and ethnic groups living and working in the United States. In this section, we provide an overview of the issues in managing a diverse workforce. Once you have read this section and completed an assessment of your staff, you should then read about the specific cultures of groups represented on your staff by using the Internet.

It is important to understand the concept of *cultural competence*, which is defined as a set of congruent behaviors, attitudes, and policies that come together in an organization or among professionals that enables people to work effectively in cross-cultural situations. It is the willingness and ability of the organization and the managers to value the importance of culture in managing a diverse workforce as well as in the delivery of services to all segments of the population. The word *culture* is used because it implies the integrated pattern of human thoughts, communications, actions, customs, beliefs, values, and institutions of racial, ethnic, religious or social groups. The word *competence* is used because it implies having a capacity to function effectively by learning new patterns of behavior and effectively applying them in the appropriate settings (Cross, Bazron, & Isaacs, 1989).

The five essential elements that contribute to an organization's ability to become more culturally competent are:

- Valuing diversity by accepting and respecting differences.
- Performing a cultural self-assessment.
- Being conscious of the "dynamics" inherent when cultures interact. Many factors can affect cross-cultural interactions such as historical cultural experiences, differing religious beliefs, and family structures and values, to name a few.
- Learning and gaining knowledge about culture and cultural dynamics. The learning then must be integrated into every facet of the human resource model from selection, development, and evaluation. All staff must be trained in issues of cultural diversity. Many health care organizations have done

a good job in educating staff about cultural diversity and the client; however, this also needs to be done to address diversity among the staff.

- Developing adaptations to service delivery reflecting an understanding of diversity between and within cultures. This fifth element of cultural competence specifically focuses on changing activities to fit cultural norms (Cross, Bazron, & Isaacs, 1989).

Generational Diversity

A major focus in health care today is the differences in the values and needs of the different age groups working in the organization. What motivates older workers is different from (not better or worse than) what motivates younger workers. As the clinical leader, you need to understand these differences and use different techniques to reward and motivate individuals of different ages. But equally important, you need to help the staff to understand and appreciate the differences as well.

Human resource experts generally use four categories to describe the different generations in the workforce. How these categories are labeled and the range of years included in each generation varies, sometimes significantly, from author to author. We are using the categories described by Hill (2004). We caution you, however, not to pigeonhole individuals based just on their age but to assess each staff member individually.

Four generations are working side by side with clashing expectations about their work and personal lives. The first and oldest group has been called many names including the Matures, Veterans, Silent Generation, and Pre Boomers. For our purposes we call this group the *Pre Boomers*. The next generation is the *Baby Boomers*, followed by *Generation X*. New to the workforce are individuals called *Generation Y*. The differences between the generations arise because their values are different as a result of what was happening in society during childhood and adolescence when their values were formed.

In short, *Pre Boomers* were born between 1925 and 1942 and grew up during the Depression and World War II. They tend to be conservative and are not risk takers. Because they grew up in bureaucratic organizations they are respectful of authority, the chain of command, believe in hard work and paying dues, and tend to be loyal to one employer. These individuals are primarily motivated by money, recognition, security, and stability. They are technically challenged, having been introduced to technology at middle age.

Baby Boomers were born between 1943 and 1964, following World War II, during a time of great economic growth. Because of the size of this generation, baby boomers are used to being catered to in the marketplace and their values predominate. Society encouraged Boomers to think individually and be creative.

They tend to define themselves by their job, are willing to contribute to and be involved in their job, and are loyal to their organization. They are motivated by money and recognition. Historically, they have been willing to work long hours, but they are entering their senior years and may not be able to perform physically challenging tasks over long work hours. Like the Pre Boomers they are technologically challenged.

Generation Xers (born 1965–1980) experienced a change in family structures including both parents working and a high divorce rate. These workers, also called "latchkey children," are therefore independent thinkers. They are disillusioned with the values of corporate America as they observed both parents working, not living a balanced life and being stressed by their jobs. They experienced watching their parents be loyal to the organization only to be laid off or demoted. As a result, this generation is not loyal to organizations, values balance between work and play, and values learning and growth, which they can take with them to other jobs. They are technologically sophisticated and desire to be active and vocal members of the team. They want to commit to the mission of the organization and become cynical if they believe the organization is not fulfilling its mission ethically or completely.

Generation Y (born after 1981) are just entering the workforce. This group is culturally diverse. Their parents were heavily involved in their lives, and they participated in many activities from soccer to music. From this, they have a strong sense of self-confidence and are technologically savvy but crave structure. They are motivated by service to others and, like the Xers, can be disillusioned if they do not see the organization being consistent with its mission and vision.

A Model for Managing Cultural and Generational Diversity

Thomas and Ely (1996) propose that there are three paradigms used by organizations to manage cultural diversity. The same paradigms can be used for thinking about generational differences as well. The first is the *discrimination and fairness paradigm*. The focus of this paradigm is on equal opportunity, fair treatment, and compliance with federal requirements. The second is the *access and legitimacy paradigm*. In this approach there is recognition that the nation is increasingly multicultural; thus consumers of health care services are likewise multicultural. As a sound business practice their needs must be met. Therefore, a demographically more diverse, multilingual workforce will result in a demographically more diverse consumer base. The third is the *learning and effectiveness paradigm* which incorporates the principles of the first two paradigms, but goes beyond them by consciously connecting diversity to approaches to work. In this model the organization internalizes the differences among the employees and respects and values differences so that it learns and grows because of them.

Table 13.1   Diversity Assessment Worksheet

Name of Employee	Ethnicity	Age	Generation	Plans

Leadership Strategies for Managing Diversity

The first step is for you to increase your own awareness about the diversity of your staff and their different values and views of work. To do this, we suggest you do a diversity assessment using Table 13.1, which is similar to the retention assessment you did in Chapter 12. By completing the table you will have a greater appreciation of the diversity (or not) of the staff and be able to identify what strategies to employ to better motivate individuals.

The good news is that embracing the third paradigm calls for the same transformational leadership strategies that we have discussed throughout the book. Once you have completed this assessment you can choose leadership strategies that allow for a variety of opinions and insights that can emerge from the cultural and generational differences of the staff. Using complexity theory as a guideline, you can consciously make new connections among the staff.

Because of the possibility of cultural and generational conflict, setting the same high expectations for performance from everyone, stimulating personal development, being open by allowing for differences to be expressed, making workers feel valued, and having a participatory nonbureaucratic structure are all techniques to move to the learning and effectiveness paradigm (Thomas & Ely, 1996).

Some final techniques specific to managing diversity are suggested:

- Recognize and acknowledge that diversity exists among the workforce and that a variety of people from different backgrounds and ethnic groups who have different values and attitudes will strengthen your clinical unit.
- Communicate and show respect for the culture and values of others, by your deeds as well as your words.
- Listen to the views of minority workers and make sure that they are included in your formal and informal networks.
- Set up mentorship programs from the cultural and generational groups that predominate.

- Provide educational in-services on the cultures and generations represented on your unit.
- Revisit your unit visions and goals and include diversity.
- Avoid stereotyping anyone from any culture.
- Avoid projecting or imposing your own culture and value system onto others (King, Sims, & Osher, n.d.).

TEAMS AND TEAM BUILDING

As complexity science informs us, focusing on the team, connecting people, and building relationships is a premiere leadership strategy. All the leadership and management strategies in this book apply to building the work team on your unit and a team-oriented environment. However, in this section, we discuss strategies specifically related to teams you have appointed for your unit to accomplish a task or outcome, such as committees and ad hoc groups versus the generic "unit team." These can be teams that report to you or that you lead. (You can also apply the information in this section to a team in which you are a member.) Your goal is to develop a group of individuals into a cohesive whole in which the members share goals, expectations, and behavioral norms while at the same time recognizing individual differences and the unique contributions of each member. Inherent in good team functioning is trust (Sullivan & Smith, 1995).

Stages of Team Development

In 1965 Tuckman proposed four stages of team development that are still widely used today. These include *forming*, *storming*, *norming*, and *performing*. It is useful to assess each of your teams, identify the stage they are in, and intervene to facilitate the team, if needed, based on the suggested strategies.

In the *forming* stage the team members first come together to lay the foundation for the team. This stage is characterized by feelings of excitement, anxiety, and uncertainties. As the appointer of the team and/or leader, your role is to provide structure to the team by stating the team goals, appointing people to the team, clarifying tasks and deadlines, and helping define the roles of the team members.

During this phase and the next, team building exercises can be used to develop trust among the group and facilitate team cohesiveness. You can search the Internet for suggestions of games and tools that can be used.

When the team enters the next stage, *storming*, members begin to realize the amount of complicated work that lies ahead. This stage can be characterized by feelings of panic and seeing the disparity between the goals of the team and the reality of the work ahead. Conflicts become evident and members of the team vie for power and control. Team members may have feelings of incompetence, confusion, and frustration.

In this stage the role of the leader is to facilitate dialogue, build trust, moderate dissent, and guide decision making and problem solving. The team is vulnerable at this point because of conflicting opinions and emotions; therefore, reaffirming the vision and purpose of the team is an important strategy.

Norming is the stage where people get used to working with one another. Conflict and competition turns to cooperation, acceptance, and comfort in giving and receiving feedback. Team members are willing to share responsibility and trust develops. At this stage the role of the leader is to take a back seat and let the team be independent. It is also a good time to delegate more and new responsibilities.

The final stage of team development is the *performing* stage. Team members are compatible with each other and everyone is "singing off the same sheet of music." Team performance is high and the focus is for the team to be successful. At this stage your role is to monitor the team and to help only when and if needed. You might suggest new goals and opportunities and have the team reflect on how well it has functioned and how to evaluate its successes.

Characteristics of High-Performing Teams

Getting the work of high performing teams done is a complicated process that includes selecting competent people, committing them to the process and the task, assuring open communication, setting up systems to expect and assure contributions from all, managing change, and resolving conflicts.

Teams are one of the premier ways of connecting people to solve problems and design new approaches. One of the first issues to consider is who should be on the team based on their competence. You need the right people with the right skills, knowledge, and attitude to accomplish the task. Further, complexity science informs you to cast a wide net and to be inclusive.

Selecting the right team leader is also vitally important. This person needs to have the respect of others (both team members and others affected by the work of the team), have good interpersonal skills, and the technical savvy to get the work done.

To be successful, each team member needs to be committed to the purpose, goals, and tasks of the team as well as assuming responsibility that the team works well together. To achieve this committment, the members of the team must see how its work is consistent with the vision of the clinical unit and the overall organization.

A useful tool for achieving commitment and alignment is to have the team develop a team charter. See Table 13.2 for a sample. A team charter should include the purpose of the team, its goals, tasks, strategies/approach, timelines, accountabilities, and linkages (Heathfield, n.d.). The process of developing a team charter helps the team and team leader to define their expectations and begin the process of communication and trust building.

For a team to work well there must be an atmosphere of collegiality and trust which allows for open and honest communication. The team members must be able to express what they think whether agreeing or disagreeing with

---

Table 13.2   Team Charter of a Recruitment and Retention Planning Team

Team Purpose

Develop a plan to address the clinical unit's recruitment and retention.

Team Goals

- Serve as a forum for reflection, idea generation, and action regarding the unit's recruitment and retention efforts.
- Develop, implement, and evaluate strategies and tactics for recruitment and retention.
- Share best practices with other clinical units regarding recruitment and retention.

Tasks

1. Identify strategies, plans, and resource requirements to address issues related to:
   - Work demands
   - Workforce makeup
   - Growth demands
   - Budget impact
   - Infrastructure

2. Craft a document that includes:
   - A plan to address workforce needs for the next 3 years
     - Succinctly stated strategies
     - Cogent rationale
     - Clear priorities/choices
     - Resource requirements
     - Implementation considerations
   - Operational plan to address shorter term (6 months) workforce needs (same items as above, with greater detail)

Table 13.2   Team Charter of a Recruitment and Retention Planning Team (*continued*)

Approach

1. Assure full understanding of issue areas and current strategies being employed.
2. Generate all possible alternatives to address the issues.
3. Research and assess the alternatives and document benefits, requirements, risks, timeframes, etc.
4. Identify decision criteria and rank strategic alternatives after assessed.
5. Conduct a financial assessment of the top ranked strategies—requirements and impact.
6. Integrate work into a final plan that clearly identifies short-term work from longer term.
7. Review and revise final draft plan and recommend for endorsement by senior leadership.

Timeline

February to June for completion of plan

Accountabilities

- The team is accountable to the clinical unit manager. Progress reports will be provided, and feedback will be sought, at least monthly.
- Clinical unit manager will periodically provide progress reports to, and seek feedback of, the director of inpatient services and the vice president of patient care services.

Linkages

- The task force members in assessing strategic alternatives will:
  - Seek input from members of the clinical unit, the director of inpatient services, and the human resources liaison.
  - Seek assistance and input of others not on the task force, as needed.

Acknowledgment: Template developed by Karen Drenkard, Vice President/ Nursing and Chief Nurse Executive, Inova Health System, Falls Church, Virginia.

---

other members of the team. People need to feel safe, be able to admit to what they do not know or cannot do, and ask for help when needed. The team members should feel comfortable in giving and receiving both positive and negative feedback. During the forming stage of the team, having a conversation about communications and what the norms of behavior are can begin to provide this atmosphere.

Successful teams encourage everyone to contribute to both the process of the team and completing the task(s) of the team. To do this each team member must have input into the discussion, be part of the decision making, and perform the work/tasks. Having one or several people predominate is destructive to effective team performance, can lead to burn-out of the people shouldering most of the responsibility, and turn off the others on the team. Members of the team must keep their promises and complete their work as agreed upon on time with the task completed accurately.

Managing change and resolving conflicts are basic skills needed for high-performing teams. The conflict management section of this chapter and the change section in Chapter 5 can be used to help analyze and resolve team conflicts and manage change.

Role and Responsibilities of the Clinical Unit Manager

When you first form a team to accomplish a specific task, your role is to set expectations, define the purpose of the team, and specify the expected outcomes. At that time you also need to tell team members what the limitations are. For instance, will there be additional money or does the outcome need to be budget neutral.

As the work of the team progresses, you need to be available for support and advice. You should receive and review progress reports and/or minutes of meetings from the team at a predetermined time. You should always be aware if the team is faltering and intervene when needed. Providing adequate resources of time and money is also essential. When the work of the team reaches a milestone or is completed, the members of the team and their accomplishments should be recognized and rewarded.

COMMUNICATIONS

In this section we look at communications from the perspective of the role and responsibilities of the clinical leader. As a health care professional you should already have an understanding of basic communication theory. Communication is a skill that involves constructing and delivering a message to someone, then listening and processing the response of the other person. This process continues back and forth. Verbal communication is strongly influenced by the tone of voice and the nonverbal communications of both parties. You can review communication theory and strategies from one of your foundational texts if needed.

From the perspective of your role as a clinical leader, you will need to consider why you need to communicate, what to communicate, when to communicate it, to whom to communicate what, and how to do it. This last skill involves assertive verbal communication, writing ability, and active listening.

Communicating and listening are not really difficult skills. Leaders who fail to communicate most often fail not because of the skill set they possess but because they have not taken the time to communicate. Communicating often gets left to do after the more concrete tasks are accomplished—the budget done and the evaluation written—and thus it does not get done. As Baldoni (2004, p. 24) states, "Communication requires discipline, thought, persever-ance, and the willingness to do it again and again every day."

Why Communicate?

Communication is important to the success of your clinical unit for many rea-sons. It is an essential tool for actualizing transformational leadership strategies. First, it is the way to reinforce the mission and vision of the unit and the organiza-tion. Second, it builds trust when you communicate with openness, integrity, and honesty. Further, well-done communication motivates staff and increases self-esteem if the leader communicates expectations and rewards performance. As we have repeatedly seen, people cannot connect, learn, and grow without suffi-cient, timely information about the external and internal environment, the strate-gic direction of the organization, change initiatives, new policies, and so forth.

What to Communicate

There is no formula to help you decide what to communicate and what not to communicate. It is certainly easier to identify what you cannot divulge such as confidential information of either a personal or personnel nature. When you have been told not to disclose organizational information (both bad news and good) until it is announced officially, you must honor that request to demonstrate that you can be trusted by your boss and others. Of course, spreading harmful gossip is never appropriate. Beyond that you will need to make a determination and use your discretion as to what you will or will not communicate. We suggest that given an option you err on the side of communicating more not less.

When to Communicate

This decision also involves much discretion and reflection on your part. If you get feedback from your staff that they are the last to know things or that they have gotten information from another source that should have come from you, that is a good indication you are not communicating in a timely fashion.

Further, communicating something only once is not enough. The key to successful communication is to sustain the communication and "stay on message." This does not necessarily mean being repetitious, using the same words and examples, but rather repeating the same themes with fresh ideas and stories (Baldoni, 2004).

To Whom to Communicate

Determining who needs to know what information is a skill. You should always be aware that in a large organization, such as your unit and health care facility, once a few people know something it moves quickly through the informal network and shadow system. Again, you should adopt a philosophy of communicating as much information to as many people as you can.

How to Communicate

Your next decision is how to communicate, in writing or verbally and individually or to a group. There is a plethora of tools used to communicate in writing including e-mails, newsletters, memoranda, bulletin board postings, communication books, and so forth. We suggest you use one or more of these techniques. Verbal communications may be one-on-one or through group meetings that range in size, composition, and leadership.

One the most common communication mistakes is using the wrong form of communication, most commonly sending an e-mail or written memo when the issue should be dealt with face to face. Written communication should not be used to give negative feedback about performance issues, to deliver "bad news," to discuss personal issues, or to resolve conflicts. All these issues have an underlying need to communicate warmth and support which is best done verbally.

A second communication mistake, whether written or verbal, is giving unclear directions and requests for action (Dumaine, 2004). In this case the clinical manager is unclear about expectations, who is responsible for what tasks, and what timelines are expected. Compare the following messages that could be either verbal conversation or written e-mail:

Unclear message: *"As a result of our lower score on the recent patient satisfaction survey, I am requesting that you read the report and be prepared to discuss it with me."*

Clear action-driven message: *"As a result of our recent decline in patient satisfaction with the noise level at night from 95% to 80%, I am requesting that all staff who work on the night shift review the report and come to our staff meeting on July 14 at 7 am with one idea to decrease the noise level."*

Similarly, in the haste of the day or the short time frame of a meeting, there is a tendency to cover too many topics at one time, whether it is in an e-mail, face to face, or in a meeting. We suggest when composing an e-mail that you keep to one topic per e-mail versus sending long e-mails with many topics. Likewise, when communicating verbally and preparing meeting agendas be sensitive to how much information you give at any one time.

Another common error is that communication of ideas is not done strategically. As we discussed in the visioning chapter, you must consistently link behaviors and decisions to the vision. This should be done both in your written and verbal communications. For example, the above message could be further strengthened by concluding with a statement such as:

"I know that you are all as concerned about this as I am, given our unit vision to be the best clinical unit in the organization!"

Verbal Communications

Verbal communications can be categorized as assertive, passive, or aggressive. As the clinical unit manager, your goal is to use assertive communication.

Assertiveness springs from self-confidence and self-esteem. It is an attitude about yourself, backed up by effective communication, that you have the right to your values and beliefs and a right to express them. Further, you need to have high esteem for others and respect their rights as well.

Assertiveness is the ability to express your thoughts, feelings, and beliefs in a direct, honest, and respectful way without violating the rights of others. The goal of assertive communication is to work toward a win-win solution to problems. Assertive people can effectively influence others by listening and negotiating so that everyone in the situation is willing to work toward a solution. The advantages of assertive communication are that it increases your feelings of self-confidence, gains you the respect of your colleagues, improves relationships, and increases trust.

Aggressive communication involves expressing thoughts, feelings, and beliefs in an inappropriate way that violates the rights of others. It means being disrespectful by putting your own wants and needs above others. When being aggressive, you attempt to get your way by not allowing others to have input or express their opinion. You are also using aggressive communication when you blame people, "bully them into your way of thinking," are disrespectful, or say harmful, hurting things.

Passive communication is when you do not express your thoughts, feelings, and beliefs. When communicating passively, you allow the needs, opinions, and judgments about others to become more important than your own. It demonstrates a lack of self-respect for your own needs, violates your own rights, and communicates a message of inferiority. When you use passive communication techniques, you are likely to have decreased self-esteem and be stressed and angry.

Assertive Communication Techiques. The premier assertiveness technique is to use "I messages." An example of such a message is "When you arrive late to work, I am angry because it delays the first patient visit of the day and puts us behind schedule."

"I" messages include three parts:

- The behavior, which tells the other person exactly what he has done or is doing. In the example this is "arriving late to work."
- The feeling—the effect that the person's behavior has on you. In this message the speaker is feeling "angry."
- The effect—what is happening because of the person's behavior. In the example the effect is "delays the first patient visit of the day and puts us behind schedule."

Following are other assertive communication techniques that you can use:

- Use factual descriptions rather than judgmental statements.
- Be clear about what you feel, what you need, and how it can be achieved.
- Been able to communicate calmly without attacking another person.
- Being able to say no when you mean no.
- Being able to give and receive positive and negative feedback.
- Be aware of your facial expressions and maintain good eye contact.
- Keep your voice firm but pleasant.
- Pay careful attention to your posture and gestures.
- Listen and let people know you have heard what they say.
- Ask questions for clarification (BUPA's Health Information Team, 2004).

Writing Skills

Writing is an important skill that often gets overlooked in management texts and leadership development programs. Being able to communicate in writing has always been an important skill, but is even more important today as we rely so heavily on e-mails. Whether you like it or not, your writing skill is often a reflection of your intellectual talent and abilities.

Obviously, we cannot teach you how to write, but we do encourage you to get feedback about your writing from your mentor. This may or may not become a professional development goal for you. We offer the following suggestions to strengthen your writing techniques.

Write and rewrite. No one writes a "perfect" memo, report, evaluation, or e-mail in one draft, so do not expect to do this. You should expect to write a minimum of four drafts. The first draft is to get your ideas and thoughts down on paper. In the second draft you organize what you have written, adding, deleting, and revising. When this is completed, you should reread what you wrote. Focus on the content to see whether you said what you wanted to stay. Last, reread and correct spelling and grammar. There are two reasons for reviewing for grammar and spelling last. First, it is almost impossible to read a document for content and grammar/spelling at the same time. Second, you are wasting time to edit grammar and spelling before the final draft, as you might be deleting sentences and paragraphs during the revision process.

Active Listening

So far we have discussed what you should do to communicate verbally and in writing. Next we need to consider the equally important skill of listening. It is through listening that you learn about your staff and about the organization. If you don't listen, you will not know what is going on, a "fatal" error for a leader.

Baldoni (2004) suggests that you need to switch your mind set to view listening as an active process, equally active as speaking. This means taking time to listen, allowing everyone to talk, and having an environment that encourages and recognizes openness of expression. To do this you must be present and visible to the staff. Listening is not a difficult skill as long as you do it sincerely, take action on what you hear when you can and if appropriate, and engage in both communicating and listening regularly.

SCENARIO

Richard is the clinical unit manager of a 30-bed inpatient oncology unit. After conducting a work analysis and based on one of the goals of the nursing department, he would like to have the patient care assistants (PCAs) learn how to draw blood. In the initial discussions of this change, an ongoing conflict between the RNs and the PCAs has exacerbated.

To resolve the conflict and to make the change, Richard feels that a strategy of collaboration is best. In analyzing the source of the conflict, Richard came up with the following:

- One group of RNs has frequently and consistently complained about the PCAs. The RNs do not feel the PCAs are qualified to do some of what they are already assigned to do, so are reluctant to delegate tasks. They are opposed to adding another skill. They are often heard to say that their license is in jeopardy or the patient could have a negative outcome if something goes wrong.
- There is another group of RNs who work well with the PCAs and are accepting of the proposed change.

- The PCAs believe that many of the RNs don't trust them. Although most are willing to learn the new skill, they believe this new responsibility will cause further conflict and mistrust.

Richard believes that due to the nursing shortage and the need to have nurses perform higher level clinical skills that this is not only an acceptable change but a very positive one for the unit. This puts Richard in direct conflict with one of the groups of RNs and most of the PCAs.

After examining the ongoing conflict between the RNs and the PCAs, Richard believes it is a result of cultural and intergenerational diversity on the unit and different perceptions of productivity. For the most part the PCAs are between 40 and 50 years old and are African American. The RNs are primarily Caucasian with a few Hispanic nurses. Their age ranges from 20 to 62. Both the RNs and PCAs generally believe the other group is not working hard enough or is willing to help each other out.

Richard has talked with his immediate supervisor and the hospital Education Department. He has also reviewed the state law and discussed this with his peers in the organization and externally.

Richard decides to set up and lead a meeting of representative members of the RNs and PCAs. At the first meeting he set up ground rules for how the meeting would be organized. To assure that everyone would have an opportunity to speak, he would go around the table and ask each person to state her view of the projected change and what she believed to be the pros and cons of the change. He asked that they all listen closely to each other and to suspend reaction or comment until the end. After this he expressed his own opinion and explained why he felt the change was needed. At the end of this round table, he then asked the group to compose a master list of pros and cons that-represented the thinking of everyone in the group. At the end of the meeting he commented on how well the group had worked together and what great contributions everyone had made. He shared his analysis of the diversity and productivity conflicts on the unit and asked everyone to consider how these differences could affect the group's tasks.

Two weeks later he reconvened the group. After asking each person how they now felt, he realized that there had been a small change of opinion and that people were more willing to develop a plan to implement this change. Several members of the group discussed the cultural diversity issue raised by Richard, and they supported his analysis. After several more meetings the group reached a consensus that included the following:

- The PCAs would be trained to draw blood by the Education Department.
- RNs would assume responsibility for observing the PCAs draw blood for the first five times they were assigned the task. A flow sheet would

be developed to document this so that everyone on the unit was comfortable with the skills of each person and would trust the PCAs to perform the task.

- The PCAs would provide an in-service to the RNs during Black History Month related to the contributions of African Americans to health care. They decided to bring a selection of ethnic foods to this meeting.
- One of the baby boomer nurses and one generation X nurse would provide an in-service for the unit on intergenerational diversity. They planned to dress appropriate to the times when they were teenagers.

SCENARIO ANALYSIS

When viewing this scenario through the lens of transformational leadership, we see two major transformational leadership strategies in play. The first is building trust among the team. Richard helped to build trust by pulling together a group, setting expectations for how the people would behave with one another, and by sincerely listening to everyone. The group has a history of mistrust: the RNs doubt the skills of the PCAs and thus worry about their license and patient outcomes; the PCAs know that this mistrust exits, so they distance themselves from the RNs and are reluctant to share mistakes or admit what they don't know. The short-cycle feedback loop (see Chapter 2) is now rolling! What Richard has attempted to do is open up communication and sharing of feelings and beliefs as a first step. Another source of organizational trust is believing the person is competent to do the task. Having the PCAs trained and observed drawing blood will further increase trust. Eventually this may transfer to trusting them about their competencies in other skills.

The second transformational leadership strategy is building self-esteem. Richard set high expectations that the group could find a solution. He addressed the cultural and generational diversity issues head on and asked that they be surfaced and discussed. From this, in-services were set up to begin to increase diversity understanding.

Using the principles of Leadership IQ, Richard is assuming the role of connector, healer, and protector. As a connector, Richard built and enhanced relationships among a targeted group of individuals and enhanced their communication. He has designed healing strategies for the work group that had underlying conflicts. As protector, he diagnosed and responded to the threat of organizational well-being by assessing the situation and adopting conflict management strategies.

Complexity science informed Richard *that* one of his first jobs was "sense maker" and to answer the "why" question. He did this after allowing everyone to speak so as not to intimidate others or to seem to control the outcome. Further, although he might have delegated this task to someone else, because of the underlying conflict, he personally lead this effort to be present for the staff. Further, the staff chose some strategies to have fun in the in-services by serving food and wearing costumes.

Complexity science also informs us that this is only one of multiple actions that Richard must take to build trust and to resolve the ongoing conflict. This is the beginning, not the end.

APPLICATION EXERCISES

1. Think about a conflict you are currently having and choose one of the five conflict management strategies to resolve it. Ask yourself how important is the outcome of the situation and the relationship with the others involved in the conflict.
2. Using Table 13.1 conduct a diversity assessment of your staff. Once you have completed it think about where conflicts between the generations and different racial/cultural groups may arise and develop strategies to address the potential conflicts.
3. Conduct an Internet search to gain a better understanding of the different values and beliefs among the cultural and generational groups represented on your unit.
4. Have a discussion with your mentor about your communication style and how assertive you are. If you need to work on assertiveness, take a class. This is one topic best done in a setting where you can practice and get feedback.

REFERENCES

Baldoni, J. (2004). Powerful leadership communication. *Leader to Leader, 32*, 20–24.

BUPA's Health Information Team. (2004, April). *Improving assertiveness.* Retrieved May 5, 2005, from http://hcd2.bupa.co.uk/fact_sheets/html/improving_assertiveness. html

Cross, T. L., Bazron, B. J., & Isaacs, M. R. (1989). *Towards a culturally competent system of care: Vol. I.* Washington, DC: National Technical Assistance Center for Children's Health, Georgetown University Child Development Center.

Dealing with Conflict. (n.d.). Retrieved April 7, 2005, from http://www.nsba.org/sbot/ toolkit/Conflict.html

Dumaine, D. (2004). Leadership in writing: Best practices and worst mistakes. *Training and Development Magazine, 58* (12), 52–54.

Heathfield, S. M. (n.d.). *Twelve tips for team building: How to build a successful team.* Retrieved May 4, 2005, from http://humanresources.about.com/od/involvementteams/a/twelve_tip_team_2.htm

Hill, K. S. (2004). Defy the decades with multigenerational teams. *Nursing Management, 35* (1), 33–35.

King, M. A., Sims, A., & Osher, D. (n.d.). *How is cultural competence integrated in education?* Retrieved April 21, 2005, from http://www.cecpair.org/cultural/Q_integrated.htm

Masters, M. F., & Albright, R. R. (2002). *Conflict resolution in the workplace.* New York: American Management Association.

Sullivan, D. T., & Smith, A. E. (1995). Effective team building in the emergency department. *Critical decisions in emergency medicine 9,* 153–162.

Thomas, D. A., & Ely, R. J. (1996). Making differences matter: A new paradigm for managing diversity. *Harvard Business Review, 74* (5), 79–90.

Zoglio, S. W. (2005). *7 keys to building great work teams.* Retrieved May 4, 2005, from http://www.stickyminds.com/sitewide.asp?ObjectId=2769&Function=DETAILBROWSE&ObjectType=ART

CHAPTER 14

Marketing Initiatives

Michael J. Emery

To develop innovative products and services that meet needs of existing and potential customers and participate in the promotion of those services.

─────── **CHAPTER QUESTIONS** ───────

1. As a clinical manager, what is my role in marketing of my institution or service?
2. In what ways is the "market" for my clinical service different or more specific than the market for my institution?
3. What groups of individuals represent my market? Are their needs/expectations different?
4. How does my market perceive the products and services that we provide now? Is it accurate? Is it acceptable?
5. How do I want the products and services of my clinical unit to be known to others?

INTRODUCTION

Peter Drucker, one of the best-known authors of modern management principles, describes today's business enterprises as having only two functions: marketing and innovation (Drucker, 1982). While this may seem a rather narrow view and not particularly relevant to health care, it is worth considering as we examine the role of marketing initiatives that are appropriate and necessary at the level of the clinical manager in health care.

Marketing includes (1) identifying those people who could or should use our products and services, and (2) removing barriers so that use can be easily achieved. In Drucker's language, it is about "creating customers," but in the context of health care it is perhaps more about identifying people who could be using our services and products, and then turning that potential user into an actual user. If we think of marketing clinical services in this way, it seems very appropriate that as clinical managers we are involved in identifying those who need our services and then working to make access to that service as easy as possible.

Drucker's second function of any business enterprise is *innovation*. This means finding or creating new and better services, as well as new and better ways to deliver those services. Innovation leads to the "what" of marketing and suggests that we must know our products and services well, be able to describe them to others, and be looking for opportunities to improve current products and services, as well as develop new ones. Innovation is identifying a consumer need and then serving that need in a better way.

MARKETING PRINCIPLES

Principles of marketing are numerous and vary from simple to complex, and generic to very specialized. Marketing principles, however, tend to be organized around three themes: those addressing the consumer, the product, and the message (Iacobucci, 2001). Consumer themes address who the consumers are, what segment of the population they represent, and how their needs or demands are expressed. They are the target of marketing and so must be understood in regard to the size, characteristics, and expectations of the consumer group. The product theme addresses issues of both what the product or service is and how the product or service is known or understood. That is, What is the reputation or the brand of product or service? These themes focus on the description of the product or service from the consumer's perspective, not the producer or provider's perspective. That is to say, how do people who use the service or product describe it, rather than how does the provider of the service or product describe it. Finally, the theme having to do with the message addresses how to speak to potential consumers and what we say to them. This theme focuses on the notion of a promise or commitment, the trust developed by consumers, and the evidence upon which we base our promises within the marketing process. These three aspects of marketing encompass then the majority of the marketing literature: knowing the potential consumer, understanding the product or services, and linking the message about the product or service to the needs or wants of the prospective consumer.

Marketing is a motivational process. It depends on the successful motivation of a consumer to seek out, prefer, select, or otherwise demand a particular service or product (Hoyer & MacInnis, 2000). Successful marketing, as Drucker says, makes potential consumers actual consumers. The consumer must be motivated to select a product or service through the marketing process. Of course, having a good and useful product or service to offer makes marketing much easier, but good and useful products and services don't necessarily market themselves. The link between consumer, product or service, and message must still be made.

SUCCESS IN MARKETING

Success in marketing is based on six elements of the marketing process. Each is important, although we can see greater relevance to health care marketing in some of these elements more than others. The successful marketing plan must include productivity, innovation, access, alliances, globalization, and quality (Magrath, 1992).

Marketing must be *productive* in the sense that it creates new consumers or promotes the consumption of more products or services. Marketing efforts require financial resources and these expenses must at least be offset by an increase in revenues that will support the marketing effort. *Innovation* is required both in the identification of new products and services as well as how to present them. The message to be presented must be new, different, or unique to be effective. *Access* to potential consumers of new products or services allows them to become actual consumers. This means that the product or service must be easy to find, available, and convenient to use. *Alliances* suggest that most products and services reach the consumer through the efforts of several individuals or groups responsible for creating and delivering the product or service. These groups must be well coordinated and work well together to get the product or service to the consumer. *Globalization* may seem an odd notion in terms of health care marketing, but this really suggests getting the product or service to the widest available group of consumers. In health care this may mean satellite services, traveling clinical resources, later or early hours of service, and transportation systems for consumers and other such resources to make health services and products available to the widest possible consumer group. *Quality* is closely related to patient satisfaction, effectiveness, and good communication. While quality is most often subjective and determined by consumers, it will likely be very influential in the ultimate success of marketing efforts (Table 14.1).

MARKETING STRATEGIES

Some marketing strategies are more likely suited to health care products and services. We have all seen examples of health care marketing that seems a little too slick, often heavy on making a customer out of everyone/anyone, and light on explaining the innovative services and products that are available. The ethics of marketing is and should be different for professional services as professional people have a fiduciary responsibility to serve as the client's advocate or

Table 14.1 Six Imperatives of Marketing

Productivity
- Increase sales
- Increase market share
- Reduced cost of products and services through volume

Innovation
- New products and services
- Better branding of products and services

Access
- Availability
- Convenience
- Easily located

Alliances
- Collaboration within the organization
- Partnerships external to the organization

Globalization
- New markets
- Mobile services
- Expanded hours of service
- Transportation to products and services

Quality
- Patient satisfaction
- Effective products and services
- Good communication

Source: Magrath, A. J. (1992). *The six imperatives of marketing.* New York: American Management Association.

representative, as compared to the marketing ethics of "buyer beware" that governs some marketing efforts (Nosse & Friberg, 1992). That being said, it is important to consider the appropriate role of marketing within our clinical units and facilities because it means communicating better and more clearly with our would-be consumers about the innovative products and services that we have developed to serve them. To begin to consider how best to market our clinical units to would-be consumers, we need to ask several questions:

- Who are my consumers?
- What are the services and products my unit provides?

- How are we currently "known" by our consumers?
- Who is our competition?
- What are the best/most acceptable ways to promote our services/products?

Who Are Our Consumers?

Taking these questions in order, let's think first about who our consumers are. Clearly, there are several customer groups, so as we think of marketing we are likely to be marketing to more than one group of consumers that have different needs and expectations. (See Chapter 8 for additional discussion of the consumer groups.) For example, our patients or clients are clearly our consumers but perhaps also their families, as well as those who request or order our services (such as physicians, nurse practitioners, physician assistants, and so on). Our consumers likely also include the general public when our services relate to public health or health education. Our student professionals are our consumers as well, when we think about the role we play in recruitment and retention of staff. Clearly, these various groups have different needs, expectations, and priorities that we may elect to include in a marketing plan. It may also be useful to think about who are our primary consumers; that is, who do we serve first? Most often we think of patients here, and clearly they are a primary consumer. But if our services are primarily referral or prescription based (such as imaging, pharmacy, laboratory services, and rehab services), then another primary consumer may be the persons or groups who request or order our services (Knight, Infrastructure . . . , 1998).

What Are the Services and Products My Unit Provides?

Next, what are the services or products my clinical unit provides? The answers may seem obvious, but it is often useful to list or describe these services and products. First, there are most likely several distinct services and products. Can we describe each distinctly? What does it include? When does it begin and end? Is it separately recognizable by the consumers? In health care it is sometimes difficult to think about "separate" services or products that we provide, but health care billing procedures clearly separate and distinguish one service or product from another. This gives you some insight into the way others see your services and products. Are these descriptions of services and products appropriate and representative? Another source of identifying services and products is in the mission statement of the unit or the organization. What do we say that we do? What do we provide? How is it recognized? This also tells us what we are telling our consumers about our products and services (Walter, 1993).

How Are We Currently "Known" by Our Consumers?

We next need to think about how our customers would describe our clinical unit. What is the reputation or "brand" when it comes to services and products that we provide. Much has been written about this recently in the name of "branding" or creating a brand name for ourselves. While this idea has been around for some time, it has just recently come to health care services, as we are increasingly expected to function like a marketplace (Keesling, 1993; Speak, 1996; Petromilli, 1999; Bashe, 2001; Smith, B., 2002; Parish, 2004; Dominiak, 2004). Reputation or brand is very important in health care, because ultimately our consumers must trust that we will provide what we say we will provide. As traditional consumers, our patients and clients are disadvantaged because they may not be able to judge our services and products themselves due to acuteness of illness, our specialized knowledge, complexities of technologies, and so on. They therefore must trust us to do what we have promised, and that is where reputation and brand become so important (Berwick, 2003; Hughes, 2003; Checkland, 2004; and Urban, 2004). Our brand (our public promise and our reputation) must drive our marketing, not vice versa. Otherwise, we promise what we do not have or cannot deliver and the trust of our consumers is diminished or lost. Think of some of the branding ideas present in marketing outside of health care: for example, "You're in good hands with Allstate" (auto insurance) and "GE—we bring good things to life." Do these slogans allow these companies to stand apart from another providing the same services? Does it emphasize what they uniquely do well? Do they live up to the promise that they make? Branding can be a helpful tool if you know first what your brand/your promise is to the consumer and then live up to the promise in the best possible way.

Who Is Our Competition?

Next, who else provides the products or services that you do? Who is our competition? In many parts of our country, health care was not a service in which we thought about competition, until recently. Services were too broadly spread out. Populations of people and geographical regions were divided by provider groups so that overlapping services were minimized. More recently, however, competition has been introduced and encouraged as a way to contain health care costs and provide consumers with choice. This means that we must know who else provides the same services and products and consider how the consumer will go about choosing between two or more competing providers. Issues such as quality, effectiveness, cost, and access will influence choice when providers are in competition with one another. It is important to know these characteristics of competing providers (Smith, D., 2004).

Assessing our competing health care providers allows us to look for gaps or holes in the range of products and services that consumers need and demand. Developing products and services for these gaps or holes is the concept of niche marketing. Recognizing an unmet need and a consumer group that wants this is the first step. Then you can decide if you can provide this product or service and if it is appropriate for you to do so. If you proceed, you then have an identified target group to whom you can market this added product or service. As competition has increased, the importance of looking for niche markets has become more important in the strategic planning of health care organizations.

What Are the Best/Most Acceptable Ways to Promote Our Services/Products?

Once you have identified your consumers, delineated the products and services that you provide, assessed and clarified your reputation or brand, and determined who your competition is, you must think about the method(s) of marketing that will work best for you and what your message will be. What are the best/most acceptable ways to promote your services/products? What do you want to say to your consumers? What is the evidence to be used in marketing? Where does it come from? Is it reliable and accurate? As mentioned above, you must first know your reputation or brand. Now you must determine how best to get that message out to your consumers. The message is guided by your reputation or brand (what do we do well, what are we known for). Sometimes the answers to these questions are not positive (we are known for long waiting periods before treatments). In this case, we must return to the branding activities and mission statements to reassess what we say we are going to do (our promise) and then determine what must be done to better deliver on our promise. If your reputation is a positive one, then you need to think about what evidence exists to support that and how to get that information into the hands of your consumers in a convincing way. This allows you to repair the consumer trust that you may have lost (not delivering what you promised) or reinforce the trust that you developed by delivering what was already promised.

At this point it would be useful to consider the role of the Internet in consumer information and marketing. The Internet has rapidly opened up access for many people to a vast array of information sites. These sites include good, bad, and incomplete information. The information obtained is sometimes very relevant to a particular client or situation, and at other times the information is not relevant. Consumers can access this information rapidly and easily. Assessing the information (accuracy, completeness, and relevance) is more difficult and may require the assistance of you and your staff. Because information of all kinds (good, bad, and incomplete) has become so influential in marketing, it is important that you consider the information (and its accuracy, completeness, and relevance) that you have available to you in marketing your clinical unit or organization. Like it or not, health information has become one of the languages of marketing. We must be able to speak that language in a credible and trustworthy way when talking about our own products and services (Coile, 2000; Sastry, 2002).

SPECIAL CONSIDERATIONS FOR MARKETING IN HEALTH CARE

What makes our products and services marketable? In health care, marketing is most often organized around characteristics of quality, effectiveness, cost, and access (Knight, Provider Networks . . . , 1998).

Quality is most often described in terms of patient satisfaction, talked about in Chapter 8. Quality is a perception of consumers that includes how they were treated, if they were satisfied with the result of their care, if communication with providers was satisfactory, and if their providers were truthful and kept their promises. While we can attempt to measure quality or define it, ultimately the consumer determines if he was satisfied. Hence, the consumer determines the quality of the service or product.

Effectiveness is an outcome of care that is more easily measured externally by achieving intended results, minimizing variations in the intended course of care, and involving the appropriate people (patient, family, other providers, etc.) in communications in a timely way. Effectiveness is about achieving goals, whether they are for a client, for a population of people, or for the clinical unit.

Cost as a factor in marketing is not always about the lowest cost, but more about the value of the product or service. Value is the benefit received in relationship to cost. Receiving significant benefit for a moderate cost would be considered more valuable than receiving little benefit but at the lowest possible cost. When cost is talked about in marketing, it is usually related to questions of fairness, value, and consistency. Is the cost fair/equitable across people? Is it equally burdensome? Is the cost in line with the benefit that the client received? (That is, was it worth the cost?) Is the cost what was expected/explained? Is the cost predictable? Also, what was the cost to the patient (out-of-pocket expenses) versus the overall cost of the service or product?

When we think about *access* to products or services from a marketing point of view, we are really asking how we make potential clients actual clients.

Creating access means removing barriers, creating ease, availability, and comfort when others use our products and services. We may not think about access as readily in health care because we are often the "only game in town," however, increasingly others will find a way to give clients a choice, and so access to our products and services needs to be as easy, quick, and comfortable as we can make it.

When we think about marketing strategies that could impact on these characteristics of our products and services, we recognize immediately that all aspects of these strategies are not within our control as a clinical manager. For example, our institution may determine the cost of our service, or determine how the client reaches us within the institution. Conversely, there are elements of each of these characteristics that can only be addressed at the level of the delivery of the product or service. Addressing the individual patient or client and their needs is an aspect of quality that can only be addressed at the interface between consumer and provider. For example, communicating well and in a timely fashion with consumers and their families is an essential part of our clinical unit's effectiveness.

ROLE OF THE CLINICAL MANAGER

As a clinical manager, you can serve several important functions in the marketing process. Indeed, you may be best suited for some of these functions as you are closest to the provision of services and products and have influence over the way in which these are delivered and by whom (see Table 14.2).

You are uniquely positioned to know and clarify the evidence that supports the unit's or organization's marketing claims. The clinical manager knows what information exists to either support or disagree with marketing claims and therefore be able to determine the need to reexamine and redirect branding activities and clarify reputation so that marketing efforts are consistent with the mission, reputation, and brand of your unit or service.

Also, you interact more than other administrators with the consumers of your services and products. This positions you to disseminate the evidence that you have to support your marketing claims. The positive outcomes of your services and products need to reach those people making the decisions to use your services and products. This makes you the source of product and service information for consumers and the "face" behind the "promise." You have a crucial role in the establishment and maintenance of trust between the consumer and the provider.

As mentioned earlier, the assessment of competition identifies overlapping services and areas of unmet need, leading to recognition of niche market opportunities. As clinical manager, you can identify opportunities for niche markets

Table 14.2   Clinical Manager's Unique Vantage Point for Marketing

Marketing Information

- Know the reputation of the clinical unit
- Find the evidence to support the reputation
- Identify disparity between reputation and evidence

Consumer Interaction

- Consumer satisfaction
- The "face" behind the "promise"
- Establish consumer trust

Niche Markets

- Identify niche opportunities
- Determine appropriateness of fit

Brand Assessment

- Is the branding correct and complete?
- Does the clinical unit deliver on its promise?

Institutional Collaboration

- Collaboration among clinical units
- Contribution of each clinical unit to the organization's mission and brand

and determine the fit with the institution's mission and strategic plans. Your input is valuable in determining if such opportunities should be pursued by your clinical unit. The pursuit of niche markets must be consistent with the mission of the organization and clinical unit. Your vantage point allows you to assess the niche market for fit within your institution and clinical service. Pursuit of niche markets also can include interdisciplinary or multi-unit opportunities that will require that several clinical managers assess the opportunity together.

Marketing succeeds or fails based in large part on our ability to deliver what we promise. The clinical manager can promote the image/brand of the clinical service or institution as a local representative within the clinical unit. Perhaps more important, however, is the role the clinical manager can play in assessing the consistency between what is promised by the institution through marketing and what is actually delivered at the interface between consumer and provider. The clinical manager has the best view of this interaction and knows first when a promise is not being delivered.

Finally, the clinical manager represents the clinical unit within the institution's overall marketing efforts. You know best how you fit into the larger scheme. What critical aspect of the institution's marketing promise does your unit deliver? How do you make it possible for another unit in the organization to deliver on its promise? What are the constraints in your unit that impact on your ability or others to deliver the institution's promise? These important questions are best answered from the clinical manager's vantage point and addressing these allow the institution to live up to its marketing promises.

Marketing is a shared responsibility and succeeds best when key players from several vantage points combine to identify, articulate, and live up to the promise we make to our consumers. The clinical managers have an important perspective because they participate in the marketing efforts knowing best the interface between consumer and product or service. As a clinical manager, you are the reality check, the "face behind the promise," and the best judge of what can be delivered and how well. Marketing is not your primary responsibility, but successful marketing of a service, product, or an institution cannot happen without you.

SCENARIO

As a director of rehabilitation services, Roger has been asked to participate as a member of a marketing team brought together to introduce a new long-term care unit in the community hospital where he works. The purpose of adding a new long-term care unit is to allow a better continuum of care for patients following surgery, for those with functional decline in chronic illness, and for patients following significant injuries. Roger anticipates that the population served will be largely geriatric patients and, for the most part, coming from the community hospital's medical, surgical, orthopedic, and neurology patient care units. The community hospital's rehabilitation service has occupational therapists, physical therapists, and speech/language pathologists. An analysis of community resources for long-term care completed by the hospital's public relations office has determined that there is considerable need in the community for more long-term care beds. This has been evidenced by a 20–30 day waiting period at existing facilities, transfer of 20 percent of all patients needing long-term care from the community hospital to long-term care facilities in other communities, and longer stays in the community hospital for those needing these services, up to 1.5 days on average.

The rehab services that Roger currently manages have a good reputation in the community for both inpatient and outpatient services. Patient satisfaction surveys indicate that 90 percent of all patients passing through the service express either "high" or "very high" satisfaction with the quality of care received, the professionalism of the staff, and the timeliness of scheduled appointments and services. Roger has helped to develop the current reputation and marketing approach for rehab services at the hospital. The branding for rehab services has been, "Expert care in your own hometown." Roger reflects on how he can best contribute to the efforts of the marketing team for the new long-term care unit.

SCENARIO ANALYSIS

Using the lens of transformational leadership, it is apparent that Roger is aware that the brand for this new multidisciplinary service will need to be a *shared vision* developed by the various disciplines that will be part of the new unit. All the disciplines participating in this new unit's development will need to have some ownership of the new vision and feel as though this has been developed collaboratively so that it is indeed a "shared" vision.

Roger may suggest that the current brand for the rehab service ("Expert care in your own hometown") be extended to the long-term care unit so that the positive reputation of the current rehab services can intentionally be extended to include the new service. At the same time Roger recognizes that a new *organizational culture* for the long-term care unit needs to be created, and it must include the other disciplines participating in the new unit. For this reason, he must balance the use of his rehab unit's organizational culture, which has demonstrated past successes, with the need for a new culture that is inclusive, yet can achieve the same levels of success.

Using the lens of Leadership IQ, we can see that Roger will need to play the role of *selector* in identifying the new staff that will bring the necessary skill and expertise and will be well suited for the vision and new organizational culture of this new unit. Roger will also need to play the role of *problem solver* as he works with his present clinical staff to apply existing knowledge and practice expertise (areas of postsurgical care, chronic orthopedic and neurological disorders, and injuries) to the unique requirements of a new practice setting (Medicare and private insurance regulations for rehab services in long-term care).

As we consider the scenario from the complexity science perspective, we note that Roger will need to recognize the importance of two related principles. First, that complex systems are *adaptable*. This new service will need to be able to flex and turn as it gets established. The clinical leadership must be willing to change with the needs of the new clinical unit and be flexible as the new service becomes established. Second, and related to the first, this new service will seek to *self-organize* in a way that will allow the system to make the most sense out of its operations. Roger and other clinical leaders must be observant of the organizing tendencies of the new unit and be willing to adjust and respond accordingly.

APPLICATION EXERCISES

1. If your clinical unit has a brand or reputation, identify the evidence that supports this. If the clinical unit does not have a brand or reputation, consider how you would go about establishing one.

2. What niche markets might exist for your clinical service or unit? Identify the consumer need, the type of service, and the methods of marketing for these niche opportunities.

3. Are there consumers that could benefit from your services or products? Identify what the obstacles are to these potential consumers becoming actual consumers. Consider how you can reduce or eliminate such obstacles so as to increase appropriate utilization of your service or unit.

REFERENCES

Bashe, G., & Hicks, N. J. (2001). Branding health services: defining yourself in the marketplace. *Marketing Health Services, 21* (1), 42–43.

Berwick, D. M. (2003). Improvement, trust, and the healthcare workforce. *Quality & Safety in Health Care, 12* (6), 448–452.

Checkland, K., Marshall, M., & Harrison, S. (2004). Rethinking accountability: Trust versus confidence in medical practice. *Quality & Safety in Health Care, 13* (2), 130–135.

Coile, R. C. (2000). E-Health: Reinventing healthcare in the information age. *Journal of Healthcare Management, 45* (3), 206–210.

Dominiak, M. C. (2004). The concept of branding: Is it relevant to nursing? *Nursing Science Quarterly, 17* (4), 295–300.

Drucker, P. F. (1982). *The practice of management.* New York: Harper & Row.

Hoyer, W. D., MacInnis, D. J. (2000). *Consumer behavior* (2nd ed.) Boston: Houghton Mifflin.

Hughes, R. (2003). From the talk to the walk. *Health Affairs, 22* (3), 189–191.

Iacobucci, D. (2001). *Kellogg on marketing.* New York: John Wiley & Sons.

Keesling, G. (1993). Brand name changes help health care providers win market recognition. *Health Marketing Quarterly, 10* (3/4), 41–54.

Knight, W. (1998). The infrastructure of managed care. In W. Knight (Ed.), *Managed care: What it is and how it works* (pp. 45–84). Gaithersburg, MD: Aspen Publishers, Inc.

Knight, W. (1998). Provider networks. In W. Knight (Ed.), *Managed care: What it is and how it works* (pp. 85–134). Gaithersburg, MD: Aspen Publishers, Inc.

Kosnik, L. K., & Espinosa, J. A., (2003). Microsystems in health care: Part 7. The microsystem as a platform for merging strategic planning and operations. *Joint Commission Journal on Quality and Safety, 29* (9), 452–459.

Magrath, A. J. (1992). *The six imperatives of marketing.* New York: American Management Association.

Nosse, L. J., & Friberg, D. G. (1992). Health care marketing. In L. J. Nosse & D. G. Friberg (Eds.), *Management principles for physical therapists* (pp. 177–191). Philadelphia: Williams & Wilkins.

Parish, C. (2004). Want to feel brand new? *Nursing Standard, 18* (18), 13–16.

Petromilli, M., & Michalczyk, D. (1999). Your most valuable asset: Increasing the value of your hospital through its brand. *Marketing Health Services, 19* (2), 4–9.

Sastry, S., & Carroll, P. (2002). Doctors, patients and the internet: Time to grasp the nettle. *Clinical Medicine, 2* (2), 131–133.

Smith, B. (2002). Brand medicine: The role of branding in the pharmaceutical industry. *International Journal of Medical Marketing, 2* (2), 188–189.

Smith, D. (2004). Performing as designed but not as intended?: Managing cultural change in healthcare. *Clinician in Management, 12* (2), 45–48.

Speak, K. D. (1996). The challenge of health care branding. *Journal of Health Care Marketing, 16* (4), 40–43.

Urban, G. L. (2004). The emerging era of customer advocacy. *MIT Sloan Management Review, 45* (2), 77–82.

Walter, J. (1993). Marketing in physical therapy. In J. Walter (Ed.), *Physical therapy management: An integrated science* (pp. 225–241). St. Louis: Mosby-Year Book, Inc.

CHAPTER 15

Financial Outcomes

Dori Taylor Sullivan

To employ financial management principles and techniques to serve as an effective steward of resources in fullfilling the clinical unit mission.

──────── CHAPTER QUESTIONS ────────

1. How does the current health care environment influence my performance as a clinical manager with financial responsibilities?
2. What financial management tools and techniques are essential for my success in a clinical leader role?
3. What are the roles and responsibilities that clinical managers have for the fiscal accountability of their unit(s)?
4. How do financial outcomes relate to the quality of care and service?

INTRODUCTION

The management of financial outcomes is the seventh and last competency in the clinical leader framework. It is the finale because it relates to all the competencies previously presented. The clinical manager's successful leadership in the financial domain is defined in two dimensions. First is the ability to use resources wisely and stay within budget parameters while delivering high-quality care or services. Second, care and financial outcomes should be considered in comparison with best practices from others performing similar work (benchmarking).

This chapter starts with a brief overview of how changes in the health care system and environment have and will continue to influence the clinical leader's financial responsibilities. The second section reviews the essential financial management tools and techniques that will position you for success in dealing with the money side of your operation. We then discuss the major roles and responsibilities clinical managers have for their units of responsibility. And last we discuss how financial outcomes relate to and must be considered in tandem with quality indicators for a realistic assessment of goal achievement.

Many clinical leaders become anxious about accountability for running the business or money side of the department, and some people decline these roles for that reason. We hope that through this chapter you will realize or reaffirm the view that a fundamental principal of leadership impact relates to the ability to direct resources to priority activities and personnel to achieve the organizational mission and goals. So, increasing your knowledge and skills of financial issues and resource allocation will assist you in performing all the model leadership competencies.

THE HEALTH CARE ENVIRONMENT IN THE UNITED STATES

Most experts would agree that the United States does not have a health system but rather a fragmented approach to dealing with various illnesses. There is a general perception that interest groups representing the most powerful constituencies (often defined as business, the insurance industry, and the medical profession) in the health care field have been successful in preventing real change in the health care system, despite overwhelming evidence that it is not working well for many people.

Harrington and Estes (2004, p. 2) reported that during the 1900s five major initiatives were undertaken to obtain national health insurance, the most recent being the Clinton health plan in the mid 1990s. None was successful. However, as the cost of health care in the US continues to increase more rapidly than the cost of living index and concern is mounting over the dramatic increase in the number of uninsured citizens, a true reworking of the health care system may be on the horizon.

Geyman (2003) described six myths that he believes strongly contribute to the inability to create momentum for dramatic health care reform. Each of these myths is listed below, and in subsequent sections we give a brief explanation of the facts disputing their veracity.

- "Everyone gets care anyhow."
- "We don't ration care in the US."
- "The free market can resolve our problems in health care."
- "The US health care system is basically healthy, so incremental change will address its problems."
- "The US has the best health care system in the world."
- "National health insurance is so unfeasible for political reasons that it should not be given serious consideration as a policy alternative."

Until these myths are widely recognized as untrue, there may not be sufficient momentum to fundamentally redesign and improve the current health care system.

Evolution of the Health Care System in the United States

The expanding knowledge base of medicine, advancing technology, and increasing use of hospitals and other health care services have combined with other factors to continue the spiraling increases in health care costs. A number of changes in the financing or payment systems for health care have been introduced to try to mitigate these effects. We provide a brief overview of the prior systems and describe newer arrangements to provide the context for why managing financial outcomes is such a critical part of the clinical leader role.

Fee for Service Payment Era

The fee for service payment era is described as the indemnity insurance and cost-plus reimbursement environment. Hospitals worked to attract physicians who would admit their patients and provide necessary diagnostic and treatment services. Expansion in insurance coverage in the 1950s and 1960s generally paid for these services for most employed workers, while Medicare reimbursements significantly covered care for those over age 65. Medicaid patients were a minority of patients for many institutions, and the reimbursement rates, although lower than private payers, were closer to actual costs. Little attention was devoted to care access issues by the mainstream populace, most of who felt they could receive care whenever and wherever they required it. As late as the 1970s, relatively little attention was paid to health care costs by either physicians or nurses despite the urgings of administrators. Hospitals and other health care organizations billed charges that were reimbursed either at face value or at some percentage of the amount, referred to as discounted fee for service.

During the 1980s interest in traditional health maintenance organizations (HMOs) like Kaiser Permanente grew and there was great anticipation of the ability to provide good care while reigning in health care costs using this model. Looking back, it is clear that insufficient focus on the demographics of the early HMO enrollees (mostly healthy young families) may have led to overzealous expectations. Nonetheless, a variety of strategies to "manage" health care were introduced, and these concepts continue to significantly influence care and reimbursement systems.

In the late 1970s and early 1980s, concerns regarding the cost of health care grew. Health care organizations, and especially hospitals, began embracing more traditional business approaches in considering their revenues and expenses, the efficiency of their operations, and their organizational structures. Responsibility or cost centers were seen as the focal points for reducing costs, leading to charging clinical leaders with understanding and managing their budgets, an often unfamiliar task.

Advent of Prospective Payment and DRGs

In 1983 a major change in reimbursement was adopted called prospective payment, using diagnostic related groups or DRGs. Prospective payment means that the reimbursement for a specified set of services is established before the care is provided. Diagnostic related groups (DRGs) were originally designed as a health services research tool at Yale University; however, policy makers and regulators jumped on this opportunity to drive accountability for costs into health care organizations, starting with hospitals. Under the new prospective payment system, hospitals would be allotted a certain amount of reimbursement for their patients according to rates established by patients' diagnoses as categorized through DRGs. Although first applied to Medicare patients only, the use of DRGs and prospective payments was quickly embraced by private insurance companies, who also increased their use of managed care plan techniques for controlling health care services and costs.

Devers and colleagues (2004) identified an additional major market and policy response in addition to DRGs that increased price competition from the mid 1980s to the mid 1990s. Managed care companies started selective contracting with hospitals and other health care organizations to achieve the best pricing and assurances of the quality of care provided. Due to their size, managed care companies had more negotiating power than individual physicians. This era also brought new payment arrangements related to sharing risk for high-cost patient stays that exceeded stated norms, also called outliers.

These changes fueled intense scrutiny of the various services and treatments and the costs associated with them in acute care settings; and, since length of stay (LOS) in the hospital is a fairly good predictor of the amount of resources that a patient will consume, LOS became the gold standard for managing care under DRGs.

An interesting dialogue that intensified under the prospective payment system was the issue of costs versus charges. Unlike many other businesses, health care organizations had little accurate knowledge of the costs of providing elements of care, and they certainly didn't have good information about the costs of a typical DRG. While in some hospitals charges for care were defined as a percentage above the costs, in most cases the costs were not really known and the charges were established through a muddy process that included how much the market would bear. This is important because without knowing the costs of delivering a certain service or caring for a specific patient DRG, the charges or allocated payment might be insufficient to even cover costs—which means the more of this service you provide, the faster you will lose money!

Not surprisingly, hospitals became very interested in managing LOSs, thus an intensified focus on discharge planning and utilization review occurred and evolved toward the current views of case management practice. Extensive databases (public and proprietary) have been created to provide comparative data for LOS and costs/charges for DRGs so performance can be assessed by each institution. Hospitals struggled to discharge patients within the suggested LOS timeframes while they also worked to more accurately estimate the costs of providing care. Prospective payment systems have now migrated to long-term care and home care settings, touching off the same types of issues and reactions as happened in acute care.

One of the most important impacts of the above change was the significant increase in patient acuity in acute care settings and, similarly, increases in sicker patients with more care needs in community settings (like home care) due to earlier discharging. This phenomenon continues today and, coupled with more stringent admission criteria and migration of care services to outpatient settings, is a major factor in the dissatisfaction of many health professional whose work volume and intensity have increased.

A second impact was the realization that little was known about the true costs of care for a given diagnosis, since each phase of care (triage, acute care, skilled nursing or long-term care, home care) was considered separately. Thus, questions were raised as to whether costs of care increased or decreased or were just shifted to other settings when considering an "episode" of care rather than just hospital costs. You may wish to refer back to Chapters 10 and 11 where the care management and quality measures for care across the continuum were presented.

This recognition and the desire to better coordinate care and control costs led to the formation of integrated delivery systems including vertical and horizontal integration strategies. An integrated delivery system or network (IDS) may be defined as an entity that "provides or arranges to provide a coordinated continuum of services to a defined population and is willing to be held clinically and fiscally accountable for the outcomes and the health status of the population served" (Shortell & colleagues, 1996, p. 7). Vertical integration refers to formalized relationships (ranging from agreements to ownership by a parent organization) of health care agencies that represent the continuum of care. For example, a hospital may have purchased or created a primary care practice, home care agency, and skilled nursing facility so that clients could receive all or most of their care with that IDS. Horizontal integration occurred as hospitals merged or were purchased with the goal of gaining efficiencies of scale as well as market clout and enhanced name recognition to promote growth and profitability. Recent research (Kitchener, 2004) has suggested that mergers have not been as effective a strategy as was touted. This activity has slowed some in the 2000s.

Reengineering and Redesign of Health Care Systems

The 1990s were also characterized by intense reengineering or redesign of patient care delivery systems and models. Major initiatives in cost accounting were launched in many health care organizations to better understand the drivers of costs and the actual costs of care for various DRGs. Knowing that in the vast majority of health care delivery settings the largest percentage of the budget is personnel, many of the reengineering efforts sought to decrease the overall number of professional staff by redistributing work tasks thought not to require professional knowledge or licensure to lesser skilled and lower paid workers. Another hallmark of this period was the decrease in management layers or levels and an increase in the span of control through loss of management positions. While processes of care delivery and support services were included and some successes achieved, the greater share of the changes were in professional roles. Norrish and Rundall (2001) noted that hospital restructuring affects the work of registered nurses in many ways. Their summary of those impacts included:

- Nurses spending more time on administration and paperwork with less time in direct patient care—a dissatisfier for many nurses.
- Contradictory findings as to whether nursing workload increased or decreased, depending upon the changes made.
- Less control over nursing work with managers acquiring additional units to lead and undermining shared governance activities and structures.

Nursing was perhaps the major but not the only discipline affected by the redesign trend. Virtually all health professions either added paraprofessional roles or increased the number of paraprofessions or support staff with the goals of better matching staff skill levels to actual workloads and, of course, to try to reduce costs. Examples in other areas include pharmacy technicians, physical and occupational therapy assistants, and social work assistants.

The early 21st century finds health care still embracing a free market approach with the expectation that competition, with some regulation, will drive down the costs of care. Private insurers and government payers have adopted stringent procedures for pre-approving and managing care in most settings, with virtually constant communication and oversight. However, under severe criticism from the general public, steps have been taken to soften the approaches to managing care through legislative actions. While the majority of hospitals and health care agencies are not-for-profit entities, an increasing number of for-profit organizations are entering the market.

The operating margin for many hospitals has rebounded somewhat from the very low positive or negative margins (positive meaning revenues exceeded costs while a negative margin means costs exceeded revenues of the 1990s), but remains very modest at 1.39 percent as reported by Moody's for fiscal year 2003. Physician practices, especially primary care, and home care agencies face similar situations. And nursing homes or skilled facilities in a number of states are in a true crisis. So the pressure related to reducing costs of care and delivering high-quality care efficiently still dominates most health care settings.

How Is Health Care Financed?

Today's health care industry consists of private for-profit insurance companies, HMOs, hospitals, physician groups, pharmaceutical companies, medical supply companies, and other health-related businesses (clinics, home care agencies, skilled nursing facilities, etc.). Most of the country has experienced significant consolidation of health care entities through the vertical and horizontal integration activities described earlier, resulting in a few larger entities. There is widespread concern that health care dollars have been redirected into for-profit entities of the industry, leaving those (organizations and individual professions) who provide care with fewer and fewer resources.

The major payer categories for health care in the US remain the government, private insurers, and self-pay (often referred to as *no pay* since the uninsured comprise much of this category). The term *payer mix* refers to the percentage of patients in a given health care organization that fall into each of these categories. With an aging population and an increasing number of uninsured, the government (through federal and state programs) is a significant if not the largest payer for many health care organizations.

Coddington et al. (1990) predicted the following outcomes of continuing with our market-based health care system, *all of which have come true in the early years of the 21st century:*

- More than 40 million uninsured
- Continued gaps in safety net coverage
- Double-digit health plan rate increases
- Small employers cutting coverage or even dropping health plans
- Increased copayments and deductibles for employees
- Large rate increases for private insurers in shrinking markets
- Numerous failures of HMOs and withdrawal from the market by larger insurance companies
- Continued cost shifting in an increasingly fragmented market
- Continued inflation of health care costs

In 2002 $1.5 trillion was spent on health care in the US. This amount is expected to increase dramatically to $2.5 trillion by 2011 (Heffler et al., 2004), consuming more and more of our gross national product each year.

Comparison of World Health System Outcomes: Do People Get What They Pay For?

It has been estimated that 95 percent of the nation's trillion plus dollar budget is spent on medical services with only 5 percent spent on health promotion and prevention (McGinnis et al., 2002). It seems clear we still have an illness-oriented system.

The US is the only country among those classified as Western industrialized nations that does not have some form of national health insurance (Geyman, 2003, p. 32). While some claim that Americans do not want a national health insurance, dissatisfaction with health care and the aging of the population are two major factors supporting a rise in general support for this concept. More and more often, people have direct knowledge of family or acquaintances who experienced difficulty in accessing or receiving necessary care. The current estimate is that there are 44 million uninsured people in the United States, comprised mainly of the poor and the working poor but with increasing numbers of workers losing or unable to afford health benefits.

It is still often proclaimed that the US health care system is the best in the world; however, virtually every health status metric—including how expensive care is—belies that claim. Starfield (2000) detailed the US ranking in health status indicators from a variety of sources and concluded that the US is not even close to being the best in the world. Some examples of health indicators showing the worst US performance were low birth weight babies and child survival at various ages; life expectancy and age-adjusted mortality; disparities in care and outcomes across social groups; and equality of family out-of-pocket expenditures for health care. The facts demonstrate that US citizens pay more for less desirable health status outcomes with difficulties related to access and coordination of care.

Implications for Clinical Managers

There will continue to be significant pressure to reduce overall health care expenditures due to spiraling health care costs as compared to normal inflation. Combined with expectations for continuous improvement and demonstration of quality outcomes, clinical leaders can expect they will need to find ways to manage or reduce costs while maintaining or enhancing the quality of care and services.

Overall approaches to managing care across the continuum and quality management were reviewed in Chapters 10 and 11. We next present the core financial management skills that clinical leaders need. We then bring the coordination, quality, and cost perspectives together as we note the roles and responsibilities of clinical leaders.

FINANCIAL MANAGEMENT FOR CLINICAL LEADERS

In this section we present an overview of financial management terms and activities essential to the clinical leader's role. While there is no expectation that clinical leaders will be financial experts, you must be confident in your ability to manage the fiscal resources associated with your areas of responsibility and understand the terminology and concepts so you can talk to the finance department staff and senior leaders.

Elements of Financial Management

There are four major elements to financial management: planning, controlling, organizing and directing, and decision making (Baker & Baker, 2004, p. 6). *Planning* requires establishing goals and developing strategies for achieving those goals. Developing a budget is the major activity in this element. *Controlling* involves assuring that the established plans or strategies are being followed, usually consisting of comparing reports of actual performance to targets. As the clinical manager, you do this when reviewing a variance report. *Organizing and directing* relate to the manager's role in using resources to best advantage. For example, clinical leaders typically establish a staffing plan (Chapter 12), then assess the degree to which it is in compliance on a daily, weekly, and monthly basis. Finally, *decision making* for each element involves analysis and evaluation to select the best alternatives for action as well as making sound mid-course adjustments when circumstances dictate a deviation from the original plan. You may have a choice of per diem staff versus outside agency staff who may cost 30 to 50 percent more because of the agency fees. Clearly, given this choice, you would hope to schedule a per diem staff member.

The field of accounting is a critical part of financial management since it organizes information for use according to a common set of generally accepted accounting principles. Financial accounting methods generate information used for external reporting to third parties so that organizations may be compared across similar metrics using generally accepted accounting principles. Financial reporting is a retrospective look at what an organization has done. Managerial accounting is for use within the organization to provide usable information for planning, controlling, organizing and directing, and decision making. Industry performance metrics as well as organization-specific indicators are provided to managers as a guide for assessment and improvement of fiscal matters. In acute care hospitals we look at metrics such as cost per equivalent discharge and hours of nursing care per patient day translated into labor dollars. In your specific areas, the indicators may relate to number of patient visits or number of procedures, calculating the revenue for those services as compared to the expenses required to provide them.

Financial management occurs within an organizational context based to some extent on the type of organization, for-profit or not-for-profit. Nonprofit organizations consist of private or government entities, neither of which pays income taxes. A common misunderstanding is that nonprofits are not allowed to make any money, when in fact they must generate more revenue than expenses to stay in business. What differs is that any margin or "profit" is invested back into the organization and its mission whereas in a for-profit company, profits are distributed among owners and/or investors. As was noted earlier, most health care organizations are nonprofit; however, there is a growing segment of for-profit businesses that own hospitals and most other types of health service delivery organizations.

Two types of organizing structures are most frequently seen in health care organizations today. *Traditional bureaucratic structures* divide functions by type and group similar types into larger reporting structures. Each functional area or department is called a responsibility center so that financial assessments of the area may be made. The terms profit or cost center may also be used. For example, in a health clinic there might be a primary care unit, specialty unit, pediatric unit, dental unit, administration, human resources, and finance. The second structure is organizing by *service lines* or major customer groupings such as cancer, cardiology, and women's health. In the service line model, all the services required by that client type are grouped so that care is coordinated and customized. You will need to understand both the managerial structure as well as the financial structure and reporting for your areas, as in some cases they are not the same model. You might report to the vice president of patient care services with the revenue from your radiology services for selected procedures flowing into the cancer center.

Managerial Accounting and Financial Analysis

We are making the assumption that you have at least heard of the financial terms we introduce in this chapter. As with other competency chapters, it is not possible for us to present a complete primer on financial management. We do seek to highlight and clarify the most important concepts and enhance your appreciation for how they fit into the bigger picture.

Basic Financial Terms

Revenue is defined as the value of services rendered, expressed at the facility's full established rates. The full rate for a chest X-ray might be $175, with one insurance company plan reimbursing $125 and another company only $110. Payments may be made after services are provided (fee for service or discounted fee for service) or before service is delivered according to agreements for care (prospective payment). These agreements tend to establish either a predetermined per person payment or a negotiated amount for specified services based on the characteristics of the group to be served. (Baker & Baker, 2004, pp. 23–24).

Gross revenue is the full "list price" value of services provided. Contractual allowances are the deductions for discounts according to the agreements in place. A deduction is also made for bad debt or the amount of money owed that is not likely to be paid or collected. Clinical leaders often work with volume of activity targets such as visits or procedures or patient days rather than actual revenue figures, but obviously these are directly related.

The term *revenue stream* refers to how money flows into the organization or its sources of business. In the most straightforward arrangement, the expenses associated with generating that revenue are considered together to get a sense of the margin or revenue to expense ratio. The margin is the positive (in the black) or negative (in the red) yield after expenses are deducted from revenues.

Expenses are the costs of generating revenue and, in complex organizations like health care, they are grouped into categories. A major distinction in expenses or costs is whether they are direct or indirect. *Direct costs* can be directly attributed to a responsibility center and tracked. For example, the radiology technologist and the supplies used to perform an X-ray are direct costs. *Indirect costs* reflect costs that are apportioned across responsibility centers to create a complete financial picture of an organization. For example, the patient billing department expenses must be supported across multiple departments as an indirect cost, but are a necessary cost of doing business. Clinical leaders should see a listing of budgeted direct expenses while they may or may not be provided with the figure for indirect costs their area will support. Table 15.1 shows the relationship among some of these financial terms.

Another way that costs are described is whether they are fixed or variable. *Fixed costs* do not change when volume of activity goes up. Rent and minimum staffing requirements are two examples of fixed costs. *Variable costs* go up or

Table 15.1   Relationship Among Selected Financial Terms

Gross Revenue from Operations	$1,000,000
– Contractual Allowances of Discounts	$100,000
– Expenses (direct and indirect)	$850,000
= Net Revenue	$50,000

Net Revenue/Gross Revenue = Margin (positive or negative)
Shown as dollar value plus as a percentage of revenue
In this case there is a positive margin of
50,000/1,000,000 = .05 or 5%

down in direct relationship to changes in activity levels. Supply costs may be an example of a variable cost when each procedure uses a prepackaged tray of instruments and supplies. A *semivariable cost* changes with activity but not in direct proportion. Staffing additions are a good example of this category since there might be a one staff member increase for three additional patients in a given setting but no further additions until there are five more patients. In general, clinical managers can, to a certain extent, control or impact volume and expense. They cannot control revenue, as that is a function of contracts with payers, bad debt, allowances, and other things that are not in their scope of influence.

Financial Analysis Statements

The financial status of an organization is expressed in four standard reports: the balance sheet, statement of revenue and expense, changes in fund balance/net worth, and statement of cash flows (Table 15.2). The *balance sheet* records what an organization owns, what it owes, and basically what it is worth (stated as fund balance for nonprofit organizations). The assets of the organization (what it owns) are equal to its liabilities (what it owes) plus its net worth/fund balance. The balance sheet is described as a snapshot at a point in time (Baker & Baker, 2004, p. 103). The *statement of revenue and expense* covers a period of time such as a year and summarizes how much revenue was generated minus the expenses used to generate the revenue, with the balance equaling the operating income. Of course, we hope to see that revenues exceeded expenses, leading to a positive balance or *margin*, often expressed as a percent of the total operating budget. However, in health care, we sometimes see operating expenses exceeding operating revenues leading to a negative margin. Some organizations offset this difference with investment income or transfers from other corporation entities like a foundation.

Changes in fund balance/net worth reflect whether an organization is moving in a positive direction by increasing its value or a negative direction by decreasing. An analogy would be that your personal savings account combined with the value of your home is a higher number this year than it was last year. If you had to withdraw $15,000 to repair your home, the number may have decreased. The excess of revenues minus expenses from operations plus any

---

Table 15.2   Standard Financial Analysis Statements

1. Balance Sheet
2. Statement of Revenue and Expense
3. Changes in Fund Balance/Net Worth
4. Statement of Cash Flows

gains from investment or nonoperations sources are added to the fund balance or net worth of an organization. Last, the *statement of cash flows* translates a variety of accounting elements including cash that has not yet been received and depreciation of appropriate assets and converts them into cash flow for a designated period. While all four reports are interrelated and important, most clinical managers would focus on the first two to get a sense of the organization's overall financial condition.

The Budget Cycle

All organizations establish a fiscal year (FY), with many using calendar years. In some states, hospitals and sometimes other health care organizations are on standardized fiscal years for purposes of regulatory reporting and comparison. At year end the appropriate financial and accounting procedures are carried out to develop the final financial reports, which are usually audited by an external public accounting firm and certified as accurate in terms of meeting required standards for this type of reporting.

The budget cycle is a series of timed activities planned to arrive at an approved budget prior to the start of the next fiscal year. Depending on the size, complexity, and culture of an organization, planning for the next year's budget might start at the beginning of each fiscal year.

A critical early component of budget planning relates to forecasting and projecting the volumes, revenues, and expenses for the next fiscal year. Forecasting and projecting may be led by finance executives, strategic planning directors, or other designated personnel. Environmental assessments, contractual changes, and trends in care needs or reimbursement must be analyzed and their relative impact estimated. These conclusions are then translated into what are called budget assumptions, the context for budget development. In addition, the identification of strategic priorities or organizational goals, along with the resources that will be required to accomplish them, must also be factored in, whether as organization-wide or unit-based initiatives.

Budget Development

The development of a budget requires several steps in addition to forecasting and projections already described. First, an approach to budget development must be selected. A zero-based budget means that each year those involved with creating the budget assume that there is a clean slate, and they start building a budget without regard to the resources allocated for the current fiscal year. Zero-based budgeting can be a useful tool for realigning expenses with changing activity priorities, but it is a difficult and labor intensive process. Most health care organizations use some variation of a historical budget that assumes most responsibility centers within the organization will continue to provide similar services, with adjustments made for volumes, new programs, and special projects.

In many organizations the budget is built by each responsibility center reviewing the general budget assumptions and perhaps collaborating to develop unit-specific assumptions if appropriate. Your role as clinical leader will involve predicting changes that would affect your unit, including volume of various services, staffing (costs and availability), equipment (needs and costs including replacement), and supplies. The clinical leader then reviews each budget line item and calculates what would be needed for the next fiscal year.

In growing markets (for example, where the population is increasing), this approach would be used more frequently since volumes and revenues are likely increasing. Using this method, the "rolled up" budget (adding together all responsibility center requests) may still exceed projected revenue by millions of dollars. The budget review process usually means a process for reducing the requested allocation to try to create a balanced budget. From your perspective as clinical manager, this approach can be frustrating if you perceive you never get what you need or request. It also leads to "game playing" and padding the budget because you know you will not get what you request so you request more than you need.

Recently some health care organizations in static or highly competitive markets have moved to an approach that we believe is more realistic. Similar to most household budgets, a projection of what the income is likely to be is made first, and then necessary expenses are factored in, followed by funding for whatever discretionary expenditures can be supported. Using this approach, there is little to be gained by having each responsibility center develop a new budget; rather, appropriate changes (adding or subtracting resources) are proposed based on projections and organizational goals. Adjustments are also made for salary increases, inflation of equipment costs, etc., usually by the finance department, after which managers may or may not review the proposed budget. While this can be frustrating, it does reflect the reality of limited resources.

Your organization may also use a flexible budgeting approach that indexes or adjusts selected budget categories based on volume or other factors during the budget year. These midyear adjustments may or may not be reflected in budget reports, depending upon the budget software system capability and magnitude of the adjustments.

Types of Budgets

Typical budgets are organized into operating budgets and capital budgets. *Operating budgets* have two major categories, personnel and supplies/equipment. Each type of expense is named and listed on a line in the budget, thus the term *line item*. In most health care organizations, personnel costs are by far the largest portion of the budget, so much effort goes into determining the necessary staffing mix, pattern, and organization. *Capital budgets* are separately created for expenditures that exceed an established dollar limit that varies across organizations. Similarly, the size of the capital budget is often determined based on what the organization believes it can afford, followed by a process for reviewing and approving capital purchases. Your ability to write a compelling justification for proposed operational and capital budget items is an important skill to acquire. Describing how a new piece of equipment will improve quality of care and decrease the professional time a service requires (and translating this information into financial terms if possible, such as a projected savings of 8 hours of professional time per week at $38 per hour is a savings of over $15,000 per year!) will be more positively received than citing that two other facilities in the area have the new equipment.

Monitoring Budget Variances

The budget variance report, as its name suggests, is a listing of each budget line item and category with the budgeted amount for the month/period and year to date; the actual amount spent for the month/period and year to date; and the difference between the two figures or variance. The variance is often expressed as the dollar difference and the percentage the variance represents from budget. Table 15.3 shows a budget variance report for a clinical area.

Clinical leaders need to analyze each line item and category, determining which are tracking according to plan and which are outliers, either too high or too low. The next step is to gather the necessary information to understand why an item is over or under budget, and whether this is a good or bad thing. If things are going better than expected, there is an opportunity to learn why and maybe extend that positive impact. More often, managers discover that lines are over budget and must investigate the causes.

There are three causes of budget variance on clinical units. These are volume, efficiency, and rate variance from the budgeted amount. Volume variances are due to more or less patient days or visits; efficiency variance relates to more or less hours per patient day, and rate variance relates to salaries (generally the use of overtime). Explanation of the mathematics to complete this easy and very helpful analysis can be found in Finkler (2000, p. 300).

In many organizations clinical managers are expected to write formal budget variance reports. These reports would identify the information just discussed along with a rationale for major variances and propose a plan for reducing the overages in various categories. Some reports also ask for managers to project expenses forward, especially when nearing the end of the fiscal year.

Table 15.3   Sample Budget Variance Report for a Clinical Area

Description	Dec 05 Budget	Dec 05 Actual	YTD Budget	YTD Actual	Variance	Percentage
Revenue						
Gross	30,000	34,000	90,000	115,000	(25,000)	(27.7%)
Allowance	10,000	14,000	30,000	45,000	(15,000)	(50.0%)
Expenses						
Salaries	21,000	23,000	63,000	65,000	(2,000)	(0.3%)
Fringe	8,400	9,200	25,200	26,000	(800)	(0.3%)
Temporary	1,000	1,200	3,000	2,200	800	26.6%
Med supp	5,000	4,800	15,000	12,000	3,000	20.0%
Office supp	800	800	2,400	2,400	0	0
Telephone	400	500	1,200	1,400	(200)	(16.7%)
Copying	100	140	300	360	(60)	(20.0%)
Travel	75	65	225	210	15	.07%

Year To Date (YTD) Budget Amounts reflect 3 months with fiscal year of October 1—September 30

Financial Roles and Responsibilities of Clinical Managers

It is now clear that for managing care, enhancing quality, and controlling costs clinical managers must have skills and knowledge in each of these areas. Focusing on where services are delivered and involving the people who actually perform the care provide the best opportunities for change and improvement. This realization has enhanced the role and responsibilities of clinical leaders, who in some organizations are seen as mini chief executive officers of their own microsystems.

As you reflect back upon prior chapters, we hope you are connecting the dots between the leadership competencies and not simply reading each one as it is presented. From visioning and strategic planning to customer needs and managing care, assessing and improving quality, promoting positive work cultures and good use of human resources, and so forth, the clinical leader must envision the desired future and systematically plan with the team to achieve that vision. The financial plan and budget are simply tools—yes, important tools to be sure—that assure that resources are being allocated and managed to produce the desired results.

Your responsibilities related to financial management and outcomes include:

- Awareness of your region and discipline's current health care environment especially related to the demand for services, reimbursement mechanisms, workforce supply, and cost pressures

- Development of projected revenues and expenses for new and existing programs within your department or area
- Monitoring and responding to budget variances
- Participating in benchmarking, either internal or external

Health care issues may be global, but the delivery of care and solutions to those issues must be driven locally. Therefore, clinical leaders must become familiar with the dynamics of their region related to which types of services for care are in demand, what the reimbursement picture is from the major payers, what the pricing range for these services is, and determination of the quality indicators and outcomes expected. While the literature may provide some general direction, the most current information will come from local sources like the hospital association and its related meeting groups, through professional networking, and from consultants.

The clinical leader's role in projecting volumes, revenues, and expenses in the preparation of an annual budget is a critical one, for it is during this process that the decisions that will affect you and your clinical unit(s) for at least the next year are finalized. Once you have a sense of the resources likely to be allocated, you can begin detailed planning for any changes or improvements that you have decided to pursue. Again, local networking along with regional or national specialty groups will likely provide the best information for program planning.

One of the most important roles a clinical leader has related to fiscal responsibility is the regular review of budget variance reports. The clinical leader's ability to analyze and take action in response to budget variance reports depends on several factors, some of which will be in your control and some of which may not. First, your comfort level in using the information presented in this chapter as a starting point for your financial responsibilities will enhance your performance in managing your budget. Second, your knowledge of your area's operations and how things are done and by whom will also help you to pinpoint issues that may be causing the variances. Third, the quality of the reports you receive in a given organization will greatly influence how well you can manage your budget.

The quality of a variance report relates to three main criteria: timeliness, accuracy, and display. Feedback regarding both revenues/volumes and expenses is essential if actions are to be taken to maximize the margin. It is of little benefit to find out three months after the fact that the medical surgical supply line item was already 200 percent over budget six months into the fiscal year. Obviously, the accuracy of the variance report is critical, both in terms of assuring that the costs assigned to your area are correctly listed (and errors do occur) and that the amount of change is proper. Finally, the layout or display of the information may facilitate or impair your ability to use the information. A logical and consistent portrayal of variance information is highly desirable. Unfortunately, depending upon the financial information systems software used, this may not be the case.

Another desirable characteristic of the variance report is that it link volumes or activity with expenses. A complaint that we hear frequently from managers is that they get variance, volume, client satisfaction data, staffing information, quality indicators, etc., but that it comes in separate reports that they must spend hours assimilating to create actionable information from a pile of data. It is in everyone's interest to work on creating and maintaining a responsibility center report that meets the needs of the organization and the clinical leaders to optimize its use. No matter how the data is portrayed, you should learn how to read and analyze the variance reports and other financial data produced by the organization.

Financial Results and Quality Outcomes

The most effective clinical leaders find ways to share financial information with the staff as a feedback mechanism. Staff with little understanding of how the finances of the unit are derived or managed will have little motivation to be cost conscious. Linking quality outcomes and care practices communicates a realistic picture that staff can embrace.

Several authors have proposed methods for assessing overall unit or organizational performance. One of the most popular is the balanced scorecard used in general business and applied to health care (Kaplan & Norton, 1996). The balanced scorecard helps us get a true sense of how an organization or its units are performing by simultaneously considering several performance domains. The original balanced scorecard includes performance measures of finance, internal business processes, learning and growth, and the customer. Many organizations have adapted these categories that are often displayed as quadrants of a table or circle. Table 15.4 shows a sample balanced scorecard for a health care organization. The point is that it won't matter much if your financial indicators are excellent if the quality outcomes and satisfaction levels

Table 15.4   Example of a Health Care Organization Balanced Scorecard

Clinical Outcomes and Functional Status of Clients	Operational Performance Indicators
Customer Satisfaction (Clients, Staff, Physicians, Payers, Community)	Financial Performance Indicators

Table 15.5   Manager Maxims to Optimize Outcomes

1. What are the mission and vision for your organization and how do you/your area's responsibilities relate to and support them?
2. Who are your customers (internal and external), and how do they view your services and products?
3. How do you measure the quality outcomes and efficiency of the major aspects of your work?
4. Is the work organized in a way that promotes quality and efficiency? How do you compare to the benchmark data available?
5. What improvement opportunities have you identified, and what were/are the results of these efforts?

(Sullivan, 1999)

of clients are poor. Similarly, if your quality is wonderful but is costing more than can be supported, the organization cannot sustain success. Benchmarking can provide valuable comparison information when high-quality information with comparable organizations can be accessed (refer back to section on benchmarking in Chapter 11). More information about the balanced scorecard approach may be accessed at www.balancedscorecard.org.

Table 15.5 lists manager maxims to optimize outcomes (Sullivan, 1999). These principles can help you to organize a holistic approach to assessing your unit(s) and deciding where the priorities for action and improvement lie, recognizing that it is impossible to deal with all identified issues at the same time.

While financial considerations will continue to be a major factor in how clinical managers lead, we cannot let it be the determining factor of how we approach our work. The approaches and tools presented in this chapter will help you maintain your perspective while enhancing your expertise in managing the financial side of your operation.

SCENARIO

A newly appointed director of nursing (DON) in a long-term care facility (LTC) was charged with analyzing the personnel costs of the operation because they had risen precipitously over the last six to eight months. Her analysis revealed two significant facts. First, there were no clear staffing standards that would promote better management and assure delivery of the established hours of care. Second, there was a significant use of agency staff to cover sick calls and personal days that were called in close to the beginning of work shifts.

The DON was equally concerned about assuring quality of care through sufficient qualified permanent staff and the financial resources being consumed through the use of agency personnel, who were paid at premium rates plus the surcharge by the agency. She recognized that immediate action was necessary even though she believed that further information and analysis would be required for a more definitive solution.

The DON calculated that assigning an additional licensed staff member to each shift would dramatically lower the cost of agency staff, help to maintain quality of care, and buy some time for her to gather additional information. She had also determined that due to a string of prior DONs who stayed in the role for short periods of time and who reportedly did not connect well with the staff, there were significant issues of trust and morale among the staff. Providing an additional staff member on each shift would convey that she heard their concerns and respected their input. The DON would also demonstrate awareness of the need to decrease the amount of money being spent on agencies by activating the plan for an additional staff member that reduced costs. The DON appointed a new staffing coordinator who was a trusted and recognized informal leader among the staff after hearing that the current staffing coordinator was perceived as indifferent to concerns about staffing and workload.

Once this plan was put into place, the DON initiated strategies to determine the issues related to excessive absences with short notice and creation of staffing plans that provided for variations in census and admissions. She ensured that staff were involved in these initiatives through surveys, focus groups, and informal conversations during unit rounds. Within five months, staffing standards were met for more than 90 percent of work shifts, and short notice absences had decreased by 40 percent.

SCENARIO ANALYSIS

The DON in this scenario was guided by each of the three main theories we discussed as part of the framework of this book. First, a number of the LIQ roles were enacted synergistically to achieve rapid improvement. Selector role considerations led to the appointment of a new staffing coordinator, to replace the incumbent who was apparently not the best fit for this important role. Second, the DON used several methods to communicate and connect with staff through the surveys, focus groups, and rounds. The evaluator role drove much of this process as the DON looked for proactive ways to address a significant problem. In her protector role she also recognized that this situation posed a threat to the organization. And last but not least she saw that healing was needed to address staff concerns about their working conditions and prior conflicts.

While not an ideal solution, the short-term actions the DON instituted were in line with complexity theory and transformational leadership principles. Increasing the involvement of the staff, "chunking" off a portion of this problem and taking action in the general desired direction, and making new connections with the staff reflect complexity principles. Sharing the beginnings of a new vision for the relationship between the DON and staff as well as building trust through response to staff perceptions and needs reflect the values of transformational leadership. As the vision is refined and even more trusting relationships evolve, the DON will increase the involvement of staff in decision making and other important aspects of evaluating care in their organization.

APPLICATION EXERCISES

1. Identify the top two services or activities of your unit. If you provide direct services to clients, what types of reimbursement arrangements or contracts are in place? Who are the major payers by percentage of revenue? If you are considered an area of indirect costs, how is the support for your operation apportioned across the institution?

2. Locate the most recent balance sheet, statement of revenue and expense, and changes in fund value/net worth for your organization. Determine what the operating margin was for the last fiscal year. Was it positive or negative, and what does this mean?

3. Review a recent budget variance printout for your department. What were the largest variances, and do you feel confident that you understand why these variances occurred. Can you calculate the volume, rate, and salary variance? Have you instituted plans to deal with the unfavorable variances?

4. Either create or revisit the balanced scorecard or quality compass for one or more of the major services your area provides. Which aspects of this assessment are meeting targets and which need improvement?

REFERENCES

Baker, J. J., & Baker, R. W. (2004). *Health care finance: Basic tools for nonfinancial managers.* Sudbury, MA: Jones and Bartlett Publishers.

Coddington, D. C., et al. (1990). *The crisis in health care: Costs, choices, and strategies.* San Francisco: Jossey-Bass.

Devers, K. J., Brewster, L. R., & Casalino, L. P. (2004). Changes in hospital competitive strategy: A new medical arms race? In C. Harrington & C. L. Estes (Eds.) *Health policy: Crisis and reform in the U.S. health care delivery system*, 4th ed. Sudbury, MA: Jones and Bartlett Publishers, 174–183.

Finkler, S. A., & Kovner, C. T. (2000). *Financial management for nurse executives and managers*. Philadelphia: W. B. Saunders.

Geyman, J. P. (2003). Myths as barriers to health care reform in the United States. *International Journal of Health Services, 33* (2), 315–329.

Harrington, C., and Estes, C. L. (2004). *Health policy: Crisis and reform in the U.S. health care delivery system*, 4th ed. Sudbury, MA: Jones and Bartlett Publishers.

Heffler, S., Smith, S., Won, G., Clemens, M. K., Keehan, S., & Zezza, M. (2004). Health spending projections for 2001–2011: The latest outlook. In C. Harrington & C. L. Estes, (Eds.) *Health policy: Crisis and reform in the U.S. health care delivery system*, 4th ed. Sudbury, MA: Jones and Bartlett Publishers, 250–259.

Kaplan, R. S., & Norton, D. P. (1996). *Translating strategy into action: The balanced scorecard*. Boston: Harvard Business School Press.

Kitchener, M. (2004). Exploding the merger myth in U.S. health care. In C. Harrington & C. L. Estes (Eds.) *Health policy: Crisis and reform in the U.S. health care delivery system*, 4th ed. Sudbury, MA: Jones and Bartlett Publishers, 162–167.

McGinnis, J. M., Williams-Russo, P. & Knickman, J. R. (2002). The case for more active policy attention to health promotion. *Health Affairs, 21* (2), 78–93.

Norrish, B. & Rundall, T. (2001). Hospital restructuring and the work of registered nurses. *The Milbank Quarterly, 79* (1), 55–79.

Shortell, S. M., Gillies, R. R., Anderson, D. A., Erickson, K. M., & Mitchell, J. B. (1996). *Remaking health care in America: Building organized delivery systems*. San Francisco: Jossey-Bass.

Starfield, B. (2000). Is US health really the best in the world? *Journal of the American Medical Association, 284* (4), 483–85.

Sullivan, D. T. (1999). *Manager maxims for optimizing outcomes*. Unpublished manuscript.

Part Three

CHAPTER 16

Achieving Magnet Status:
A Story of Leadership

Kathleen Stolzenberger
Colleen Smith

INTRODUCTION

This chapter contains a personal account of a community hospital's journey to become the first magnet hospital in its state. This story is relevant for three major reasons. First, the magnet concept itself, while defined related to nursing, reflects the goals of all positive health discipline work environments. The term *magnet hospital* was coined in the early 1980s to describe the results of research studies that identified hospitals that successfully retained a high quality and satisfied nursing workforce in competitive markets at a time when the nursing shortage was severe. Magnet hospitals were characterized by strong and participative leadership practices that enhanced professionalism and resulted in higher quality patient care. Second, the nursing leadership practices associated with creating a magnet hospital profile are derived from the theoretical lenses used in our Multi-Dimensional Leadership model: transformational leadership, Leadership IQ, and complexity science applied to health care. Third, this leadership success story highlights the interdisciplinary aspects of creating a magnet hospital, for nursing cannot achieve excellence without the participation and support of our professional colleagues. Together we create excellence!

As you read and reflect on the leadership lessons in this story you will find that the nursing magnet forces also characterize the practice of other health disciplines and are a worthy goal to seek in the name of professional performance and patient care quality.

MAGNET HOSPITAL STUDIES

The arrival of a new millennium in health care delivery has turned the international spotlight on the nursing work environment as concerns about patient safety, medical mistakes, and an acute nursing shortage continue to escalate.

Public and professional accounts of the hospital work environment describe it as a chaotic, understaffed, and intense setting fraught with the potential for error. As a result, nurse executives are eager to explore new management models that can transform their organizations into work environments that support and promote professional nursing practice.

One professional practice model gaining international attention is the American Nurses Credentialing Center (ANCC) Magnet Recognition Program for Excellence in Nursing Services. The ANCC Magnet Program grew out of research in the early 1980s aimed at identifying a national sample of hospitals with excellent reputations for attracting and retaining nurses. Forty-one hospitals were identified as "magnets" despite a national nursing shortage, demonstrating amazing congruency in organizational characteristics that were associated with their success (McClure, Poulin, & Sovie, 1983). Findings were presented as ingredients for magnetism in four categories: (a) administration; (b) organizational structure; (c) professional practice; and (d) professional development (McClure & Hinshaw, 2002). Nurse administrators were described as visionary, highly visible leaders who shared a participative management style, encouraged open communication, and supported staff nurse involvement at every level of organizational life. When asked "What makes your hospital a good place to work?" staff nurses stressed such factors as autonomy in making clinical decisions, professional recognition, mentoring, primary nursing, respect, and the ability to practice nursing as it should be practiced (McClure & Hinshaw, 2002). Nurses viewed themselves, and were viewed by administration, as accountable for their own practice.

The original magnet hospital study was a hallmark study for nursing administration. In magnet hospitals management supported professional nursing practice and strove to create the kind of work environment in which it could flourish. One of the most significant conclusions from the original magnet hospital study is the potential for modifying essential aspects of the practice environment on behalf of nurses and patients and the importance of making continuous efforts to improve it (McClure & Hinshaw, 2002).

In 1993 the American Nurses Credentialing Center (ANCC), as the accreditation arm of the American Nurses Association, established a formal program to recognize outstanding hospitals. A form of organizational accreditation, the program requires that hospitals must earn magnet designation rather than have it conferred on the basis of their reputations. Initially, the ANCC Magnet Program revolved around 14 standards of excellence for nursing services derived from findings of the original magnet study. Recently, 14 *forces of magnetism* were identified as emerging from implementation of the standards. These forces characterize a magnet hospital environment (American Nurses Credentialing Center, 2005).

Table 16.1　Forces of Magnetism

	Force	Description
1	Quality of Nursing Leadership	Nursing leaders are perceived as knowledgeable, strong risk-takers who follow an articulated philosophy in the day-to-day operations of the nursing department. Nursing leaders also convey a strong sense of advocacy and support of staff.
2	Organizational Structure	Organizations are characterized as flat, rather than tall, structures in which unit-based decision making prevails. Nursing departments are decentralized, with strong nursing representation evident in the organizational committee structure. The nursing leader serves at the executive level of the organization.
3	Management Style	Organization and nursing administrators use a participative management style, incorporating feedback from staff at all levels of the organization. Feedback is characterized as encouraged and valued. Nurses serving in leadership positions are visible, accessible, and committed to communicating effectively with staff.
4	Personnel Policies & Procedures	Salaries and benefits are competitive. Rotating shifts are minimized, and creative and flexible staffing models are used. Personnel policies are created with staff involvement, and significant administrative and clinical promotional opportunities exist.
5	Professional Models of Care	Models of care are used that give nurses the responsibility and authority for the provision of patient care. Nurses are accountable for their own practice and are the coordinators of care.
6	Quality of Care	Nurses perceive that they are providing high-quality care to their patients. Providing quality care is seen as an organizational priority as well, and nurses serving in leadership positions are viewed as responsible for developing the environment in which high-quality care can be provided.
7	Quality Improvement	Quality improvement activities are viewed as educational. Staff nurses participate in the quality

(continued)

Table 16.1   Forces of Magnetism (*continued*)

		improvement process and perceive the process as one that improves the quality of care delivered in the organization.
8	Consultation & Resources	Adequate consultation and other human resources are available. Knowledgeable experts, particularly advanced practice nurses, are available and used. In addition, peer support is given within and outside the nursing division.
9	Autonomy	Nurses are permitted and expected to practice autonomously, consistent with professional standards. Independent judgment is expected to be exercised within the context of a multidisciplinary approach to patient care.
10	Community & the Health Care Organization	Organizations that are best able to recruit and retain nurses also maintain a strong community presence. A community presence is seen in a variety of ongoing, long-term outreach programs. These outreach programs result in the organization being perceived as a strong, positive, and productive corporate citizen.
11	Nurses as Teachers	Nurses are permitted and expected to incorporate teaching in all aspects of their practice. Teaching is one activity that reportedly gives nurses a great deal of professional satisfaction.
12	Image of Nursing	Nurses are viewed as integral to the organization's ability to provide patient care services. The services provided by nurses are characterized as essential by other members of the health care team.
13	Interdisciplinary Relationships	Interdisciplinary relationships are characterized as positive. A sense of mutual respect is exhibited among all disciplines.
14	Professional Development	Significant emphasis is placed on orientation, in-service education, continuing education, formal education, and career development. Personal and professional growth and development are valued. Opportunities for competency-based clinical advancement exist, along with the resources to maintain competency.

Today applying for and sustaining ANCC magnet designation requires significant organizational commitment, dedication, and resources. The ANCC magnet Commission grants magnet status to hospitals that demonstrate achievement of magnet standards of excellence based on a rigorous appraisal process. Hospitals must submit comprehensive documentation that shows how the "forces of magnetism" are alive in the organization. If the documentation scores in the excellence range, then the organization is eligible for a site visit. The Magnet Commission votes to award magnet status based on appraisers' recommendations. Magnet hospitals must submit an interim report annually and apply for redesignation every four years. In May 2005 over 130 hospitals were designated by ANCC as magnet hospitals (American Nurses Credentialing Center, 2005). This represents only about 2 percent of American acute care hospitals.

Growing evidence supports the magnet hospital concept as a model for creating hospital work climates that support professional practice. Distinguishing characteristics of magnet hospitals have remained stable over time despite overwhelming restructuring and reengineering efforts (Aiken, Clarke, & Sloane, 2000). For almost two decades investigators have been reporting empirical associations between organizational characteristics associated with magnet hospitals and improved nurse and patient outcomes. McClure and Hinshaw (2002) summarize three waves of magnet hospital research that span two decades of study. Researchers have reported better nurse outcomes in magnet facilities: greater satisfaction, less burnout, lower turnover, and greater nurse safety (Aiken 2002; Aiken, Clarke, Sloane, Sochalski, & Silber, 2002; Aiken, Havens, & Sloane, 2000; Scott, Sochalski, & Aiken, 1999). Findings suggest that magnet hospital environments are associated with lower Medicare mortality rates (Aiken, Smith, & Lake, 1994; Estabrooks, Midodzi, Cummings, Ricker, & Giovannetti, 2005), fewer nosocomial infections and pressure ulcers, and greater patient satisfaction (Aiken, Clarke, Sloane, Sochalski, & Silber, 2002; Aiken, Clarke, & Sloane, 2000; Aiken, Sloane, Lake, Sochalski & Weber, 1999). Thus, studies suggest that the ANCC magnet hospital model is evolving as the new "gold standard" for health care organizations in search of solutions to the nursing shortage and better patient outcomes (American Nurses Credentialing Center, 2005).

SETTING FOR OUR STORY

Middlesex is an acute care community hospital in southern New England that serves 250,000 residents and employs about 2,000 people, including approximately 450 registered nurses. The average daily census is around 150 inpatients, but the hospital also provides care across a continuum of outpatient services. Recently, the hospital celebrated its 100th anniversary and was named by Solucient as one of the top 100 hospitals in the country. In 2001 it was designated as

Connecticut's first magnet hospital, the prestigious national recognition granted by the American Nurses Credentialing Center for Excellence in Nursing Services.

Major hospital services include medical-surgical and critical care for inpatients, diagnostic services including cardiac catheterization, the pregnancy and birth center, center for behavioral health, home care, and hospice/palliative care. The hospital operates an outpatient surgical center, a new cancer center, and two freestanding medical centers in neighboring communities. It sponsors a family practice residency program and participates in a number of clinical affiliations with regional health care centers and universities. Education is a deeply rooted tradition at the hospital. Its 100-year-old diploma school of nursing closed in the mid-1990s.

The chief nursing officer holds the title of vice president for nursing. She reports directly to the CEO/president of the hospital and is responsible for several clinical departments in addition to nursing, including home care, pharmacy, social work, emergency services, and the behavioral health department. She was appointed to her position in 1995. Ten nursing directors work closely with her as an administrative team. Nurse managers and supervisors join them to form the nursing leadership team.

This story describes the experiences of nurse leaders in seeking magnet designation for the hospital as the mechanism for transforming the nursing work environment.

OUR MAGNET JOURNEY BEGINS

In June of 1998, at our annual nursing leadership retreat, nurse leaders began to explore the possibility of transforming our nursing organization into an ANCC magnet facility. These retreats had become a welcome tradition in our department as a time off campus for reflection and strategic planning. Colleen Smith, vice president for nursing, had invited Mary Ann Donohue, PhD, RN, from Hackensack University Medical Center (HUMC) in New Jersey, to share her hospital's experiences in achieving and sustaining magnet designation. Our excitement grew as we learned more about the magnet award and the early evidence associating nurse retention and satisfaction with magnet designation. In particular, we were impressed with HUMC's approach to the magnet process as a partnership with staff nurses. And while our community-based hospital was much smaller, our hospitals shared the organizational commitment to excellence that undergirds the ANCC magnet model. As the retreat ended, we framed our vision to achieve magnet designation and were convinced we could make it a reality.

Looking back eight years later, we recognize how naïve we were that day as we dreamed of becoming a magnet hospital. We viewed magnet designation primarily as a prestigious credential from our own profession that would validate the exceptional caliber of professional nursing practice at our hospital.

Too often, patients and families had described nursing care at Middlesex as a "best-kept secret." The magnet award had the potential to address two important areas. Nursing excellence at Middlesex Hospital would be officially recognized through the national magnet status. Second, we recognized the potential "healing powers" magnet status might foster within the context of a dramatic reengineering initiative four years earlier that revolutionized how nurses delivered care. Later we would discover a much more expansive vision of the magnet journey and status, realizing and experiencing the power of this transformative process. Far more than an award program, magnet status was to become the foundation for a new departmental infrastructure, the evidence base propelling our strategic plan, and the catalyst for action to improve the nursing work environment (Stolzenberger, 2003).

During the summer of 1998, nurse leaders committed to learning more about the Magnet Program. Our chief nursing officer (CNO) Colleen Smith, had already taken the critical first step: obtaining initial endorsement of the idea from our CEO, Robert Kiely. From an executive perspective, our leaders recognized that pursuing magnet designation would require an organizationwide commitment involving considerable time, energy, and resources. Our CNO knew that achieving magnet designation, and sustaining it, would demand widespread collaboration across departments and disciplines. At the same time, the standards of excellence that frame the magnet model were clearly aligned with the hospital's mission, values, traditions, and strategic plans. Ensuring strategic alignment of proposed department plans reflected our CNO's allegiance to the organization. She also strongly believed in the value of building essential strategic alliances before undertaking any project that had broad implications for the organization in order to ensure its success in moving our nursing department forward.

Winning CEO endorsement propelled us into action. CNO Smith and the directors who comprised her nursing leadership team agreed to investigate the magnet application process and to evaluate our readiness to participate. As nurse leaders, we understood and espoused the *forces of magnetism* that characterize magnet hospital environments. Philosophically at least, the team agreed with the premises underlying the Magnet Program. We believed in the value of a nursing organization that advanced the quality of nursing leadership and patient care; promoted education, professional development and participative management; portrayed a positive image of nursing; served both lay and professional communities; and provided adequate resources and consultation to support professional nursing practice. We knew we were already operating in an organization where nurses enjoyed rich collaborative relationships with physicians and the interdisciplinary team. Yet we still had a great deal to learn about the magnet program standards that defined and described the forces of magnetism in practice.

At that time there were only 18 magnet-designated hospitals in the entire country. Without a "critical mass" of magnet hospital knowledge, experience, and resources, we knew we were venturing into new territory with little more than our own leadership beliefs and experiences to guide the way. Fortunately, a number of magnet hospitals were in New Jersey, our neighboring state. That summer CNO Smith and a small director group visited four magnet facilities. The visits were highly productive, with administrative colleagues sharing success stories and recommendations for how to proceed. It was an energizing, whirlwind tour that uncovered several best practices that we considered a good match for our organization.

For example, we were very impressed by those hospitals that had engaged staff nurses from the onset in their journeys toward magnet designation. The application process would involve gathering evidence of excellence in nursing practice and hosting a site visit that would focus on staff perceptions of the practice climate. As our CEO had cautioned us, we did not want to "gild the lily" in our application or prepare it from an administrative perspective alone that would isolate staff from the process. In addition, our CNO realized the enormity of the project and knew that it would necessarily consume departmental resources and energy as a strategic priority. She considered it worth the investment only if staff were enthusiastic about the idea and willing to contribute to its success. Later we discovered how wise we had been in partnering with the staff from the beginning, for it was the power of the process itself that was the most potent catalyst for change in our department.

Also, we agreed with the approach taken by the CNO of one hospital who had succeeded by gaining consensus among key stakeholders before committing to the magnet process. It was important to us to adopt a similar approach by confirming support for our plan on several fronts, beginning with the nursing leadership team and nursing staff, and including medical staff leadership, other department heads, the executive staff and the board of directors.

Building Consensus: Fall 1998

While the nursing directors' group had agreed in principle with our preliminary magnet plan, some directors were still hesitant because of the work it would involve in the midst of daily operational demands on their time and energy. Our CNO was personally convinced that striving for magnet status was the right thing to do. But she wanted consensus among directors before going forward. To help them learn more about the magnet model, she arranged another site visit to New Jersey magnet facilities for those directors who had not made the previous site visit. This proved invaluable. As before, the site visit ignited the team's enthusiasm and cemented directors' endorsement of plans to strive to become a magnet hospital.

That fall, CNO Smith and nursing directors assessed their readiness to apply for magnet status by reviewing the standards and considering what they had learned from the site visits. They recognized that nursing position descriptions fell short of defining expectations of excellence as expressed in the magnet standards. Further, the department had an ineffective committee structure that did not meet magnet expectations of a shared governance system that respected nurses' voice and authority in making decisions affecting their practice. Finally, there was a need to strengthen clinical coordination and support on nursing units through a major revision in the nurse manager role. As a result, leaders took on three major department initiatives: revision of all nursing position descriptions and performance evaluations, creation of a council model of governance, and institution of a new clinical coordinator role.

Off to a False Start

Throughout the fall, CNO Smith and the eight directors began to delve more deeply into Magnet Program requirements. Anxious to move into action, they agreed to share responsibilities for interpreting the 14 standards and plotting out tentative evidence to support their integration in our department. The group called themselves the Magnet Standards Committee, and each director assumed lead responsibility for one or two standards. Each agreed to form a core team as a standards subcommittee for the assigned standards who would be responsible for completing that section of the application. The director was to become the "expert" for that standard, charged with educating the rest of the group about its meaning and relevant evidence. The November Magnet Standards Committee was dedicated to the first standard of care, assessment.

The meeting was a disaster. Tensions mounted as directors disagreed on the interpretation of the standard and differed about value in addressing the 14 standards. Normally a cohesive and collegial group, the directors challenged each other in both verbal and nonverbal ways as they struggled with how to manage the project as well as the other major initiatives they had begun to build the department infrastructure. Their stress became palpable. The meeting unveiled the real work that lay ahead as they faced the realities of dealing with competing department priorities.

Clearly, we had moved too fast. It was apparent that the directors' preliminary assessment of the standards had been naive. No one had a comprehensive understanding of the standards or grasped the distinctions among them that was needed to avoid duplication and prevent redundancy in our application. To make matters worse, it was not clear who was in charge of making decisions about how to build the application. CNO Smith quickly realized she had underestimated directors' concerns about the additional workload involved in leading the subcommittees, gathering evidence, and writing sections of the application.

Typical of her leadership style, CNO Smith scheduled a midwinter retreat to confront these obstacles. The retreat was an opportunity to pause and reflect on our decisions, acknowledge our "false start," challenge our earlier plans and timelines, and reexamine the vision we had created as the backdrop for decisions about how to proceed. Ultimately, this proved to be a very wise decision. Smith took the authoritative stance we needed.

First, she clarified responsibilities for writing the application. Kathleen Stolzenberger, director of program development, would be the sole writer of the application. As leader, Colleen Smith assessed individual strengths and talents in the director group and wished to capitalize on Kathleen's project management and writing skills. Second, she clarified that as project coordinator Kathleen would assume primary responsibility for interpreting standards, identifying and mapping out the evidence, and leading efforts to gather needed documentation. An audible sigh of relief filled the room. Directors with demanding clinical responsibilities were instantly relieved. These announcements were a relief to Kathleen as well. In defining her authority among her peers in relation to the project, Kathleen was free to lead her colleagues and move the initiative forward.

The third decision made that day was to acknowledge that we needed to slow down our magnet timelines. CNO Smith posed an important question: "Do we just want to apply for an award, or do we want to do it right?" She reminded us of our vision that had driven us as a team to plan these changes. It was an "aha" moment for our leadership group. Suddenly it was clear. We first needed to focus on the initiatives we had begun to strengthen the department infrastructure: instituting new position descriptions and performance evaluation systems, a new council structure, and new clinical coordinator roles. It took courage to admit to the tensions among us and to acknowledge that we had been hasty in our decisions.

With Colleen as our role model, however, we knew it was the right course of action. As a result, we revised our strategic goals and extended our projected date for submitting the magnet application by 18 months. In retrospect, we are convinced that we would not be experiencing the departmental transformation currently underway if we had held on to our initial vision and timeframes. The experience reaffirmed the values of honest self-assessment, accountability, collegiality, and change management that sustained us as a leadership team.

That December CNO Smith delivered her annual State of the Union address to the nursing staff. The address focused on four major changes underway in the department, including tentative plans to pursue magnet designation. She viewed it as an excellent opportunity to determine if the nursing staff was behind the project. At the end of the presentation, Colleen invited nurses who were interested in getting involved in developing the council model or in the magnet initiative to add their names to a signup sheet. She was delighted when over 50 staff nurses signed up, an expression of staff support that Colleen viewed as critical to our success.

Another important move for our CNO was to gain support from the hospital board of directors. The board fully endorsed her plans, commenting on her enthusiasm and the strength of her convictions in delivering the presentation.

**Strengthening the Department Infrastructure:
Spring to December 1999**

During the following year we made significant strides in implementing new roles and performance appraisal processes. A task force of staff nurses and managers developed bylaws for our new nursing councils that were launched at an inaugural meeting in December of 1999. The bylaws described a one-year transition phase during which we envisioned that council leadership would shift from directors serving as chairpersons to staff nurses. We understood from the literature that fully integrating shared governance took time. Successful programs reportedly took more than five years to be fully functioning. We were prepared to make the commitment. While developing the structure was the first step, we were willing to invest in developing new staff nurse leaders and in adopting new shared decision-making processes in order to produce the outcomes of excellence we desired. Four years later we would discover that, once again, we had been wise in our thinking but naive in planning the transition timeline.

Throughout the year we continued to learn more about the magnet standards and the application process. It was our intention to form a Magnet Nurse Champion Team, modeled on the examples we had seen during site visits to Hackensack University Medical Center and Riverview Medical Center in New Jersey. Nurses who had expressed interest at the annual meeting formed a potential roster. Following recommendations from their managers, Kathleen Stolzenberger invited the nurses to attend an information session to learn more about the Magnet Nurse Champion role. We were uncertain ourselves about the details of the role or the job ahead. However, we knew the risk was worth it. By partnering with the staff, we knew we would be able to prepare an application that told the real story about nursing excellence and the quality of the practice environment at Middlesex Hospital.

From the onset we were interested in monitoring our progress in building a stronger nursing department and felt accountable for evaluating the outcome of major changes underway. This meant establishing a baseline measure of the nursing practice climate as a starting point. The literature led us to the Nursing Work Index Survey (NWI) (Aiken & Patrician, 2000; Kramer & Hafner, 1989; Lake, 2002) used in many studies to measure the nursing work environment (Laschinger et al., 2003; McClure & Hinshaw, 2002; Upenieks, 2002). Following the survey, we contracted with researchers at the University of Pennsylvania Center for Health Outcomes and Policy Research to interpret our findings. We remember the excitement we felt when Dr. Sean Clarke met with us to go over our results and how we fared in comparison to magnet hospitals. "You are looking magnet," he told us. It was the impetus we needed to begin the process of preparing the application.

Results of the NWI survey included strong scores, including those for physician-nurse collaboration. Armed with the data, CNO Smith attended a round of medical staff department meetings to introduce the Magnet Program, share these findings, and recruit medical staff support for our magnet plans.

PREPARING THE APPLICATION: JANUARY TO NOVEMBER 2000

Magnet Advisory Committee

CNO Smith began the new year by establishing a magnet advisory committee. This was a "best practice" we had heard about during site visits. The committee was formed to strengthen the network of support we would need to become a magnet organization and to formalize alliances that she knew were critical to our success. Members included vice presidents, key department heads, medical staff leaders, and a representative from the board, in addition to Colleen Smith and Kathleen Stolzenberger. Undoubtedly, this committee was an important support mechanism for Colleen Smith and helped us frame our magnet journey as a hospitalwide initiative.

Nurse Champion Team

We believe that establishing our Nurse Champion Team was among the most significant decisions we made. Forty staff nurses accepted our invitation to become Nurse Champions. As our most enthusiastic and dedicated professional nurses, they became completely engaged in the magnet process. They served as staff liaisons, educators, data collectors, and cheerleaders as we carved away at preparing our application. Among themselves they shared examples of excellence from their own practice areas. In the process nurses across practice settings gained deep appreciation for each other as shared experiences began to break down communication barriers. Meetings became the forums as well for nurturing the new partnership we desired between staff and administration as colleagues with a shared dream.

Through creative use of fun-filled scavenger hunts and other data-gathering exercises, the nurses gathered evidence that gave them a sense of ownership, recognized their practice, and enriched our application. When puzzled by the standards or where the evidence belonged, nurses were encouraged to "just tell a story." This was an approach that not only uncovered a wealth of evidence but also generated a compendium of nurse stories so powerful that we decided to publish them internally. During Nurses Week that year we presented our first volume of *Nurse Stories: Voices of Excellence.* This has now become another valued tradition in our department, with volume six published in 2005.

As leaders, however, we discovered we had made one big mistake in our work with the Nurse Champions. While the Nurse Champion Team tightened relationships between staff and administration, the process was excluding managers. We had failed to keep all directors and clinical coordinators in the communication loop. Nurse Champions were busy learning, educating staff, and gathering data but their managers were unaware of what was going on. Realizing this, we took steps to correct this serious communication gap and to reinforce the importance of the staff-manager relationship. This was an important lesson that we carried with us as we planned how to sustain magnet designation in the years to come.

Writing the magnet application and organizing supporting documentation was an intense process that took almost six months. At the end of November, it was finally professionally bound and packed for shipping. Early in 2000 we received word that appraisers had scored our application "in the range of excellence," qualifying us for a site visit. The entire organization shared in our excitement.

Magnet Site Visit

Preparing for the appraisal visit was an extensive hospitalwide collaborative effort. The experience went very smoothly because of the strong coalitions of support that Colleen Smith had established on every front. Every department participated, highlighting the exceptional interdepartmental collaboration and interdisciplinary relationships that typify care delivery processes at Middlesex. Our Nurse Champion co-chairs shone as they escorted the appraisers throughout the institution. We all shared a sense of immense pride in the staff and felt their excitement grow as they interacted with the appraisers.

MEANING OF MAGNET STATUS

June 1, 2001 was an unforgettable day. The chairperson of the ANCC magnet commission called to announce that we had been awarded magnet designation. We were now the first and only Magnet hospital in Connecticut. What followed was a summer of celebration for the entire hospital community, including a beach club reception hosted by our CEO to honor the Nurse Champion Team.

That summer our nursing leadership retreat gave us a chance to review the appraisers' recommendations for our continued growth as a nursing department. Essentially, there were two recommendations: (1) to continue to develop the nursing councils and other infrastructure changes we had initiated and (2) to focus on strengthening nursing research in our department.

Earning magnet designation was an exciting but intense and arduous process. We shared immense pride in our accomplishment. However, we were in for another awakening. We discovered in the months that followed that sustaining magnet status was going to be far more challenging than achieving the initial designation.

During the first post-award year, our leadership meetings focused on strategic planning, using the ANCC commission recommendations and the magnet standards as the platform for our decisions. We scrutinized the standards more critically and conducted another gap analysis to set goals and determine new directions for our nursing department. In the process of doing so, we made four startling discoveries.

First, we finally understood the magnet model. It had taken three years of intensive work to become a magnet hospital, numerous presentations explaining the program and our experiences, and ongoing gap analyses following designation before we grasped the real meaning of the program. The standards and *forces of magnetism* suddenly became crystal clear. They served as the mechanisms for strengthening the nursing practice environment at our hospital. The Magnet Program is not a demonstration project. In fact, it is a directive for nurse leaders who want to build a better nursing work environment. Committing to it meant striving for overall transformation in our nursing department, not just instituting new roles or procedures. Instead, our department stood on the edge of change, facing a future of uncertainty, complexity, and instability that characterizes the process of real transformative change.

Second, we recognized that, while the program celebrates excellence in nursing practice, it is essentially a mandate for nursing leadership. The assumptions underlying the magnet model became visible to us. We illustrated them as the magnet formula for success. That is, in the context of a dynamic and supportive organization, visionary nurse leaders embrace the magnet model as an evidence-based framework for organizing and managing nursing services. In doing so, they create a practice climate where nurses have the resources and support they need to provide the highest quality of professional care. It is the professional practice environment that attracts and retains excellent nurses because they are empowered to provide the desired level of professional nursing care. Consequently, patients benefit from the highest quality of care.

Third, as our understanding grew, so did our sense of accountability. As leaders, we grasped the enormity of our responsibility for transforming the nursing department into a genuine magnet environment. At the start of our journey, without a clear evidence base, we had struggled to answer nurses' questions about how they would benefit from magnet designation to the staff. Answering honestly, Colleen Smith had simply answered: "We don't know—but we believe it is the right thing to do, so why not try?" Now she addressed the staff and other audiences with determination and conviction, knowing that the magnet model represents the gold standard as a framework for nursing services administration. "I believe as leaders we are accountable for upholding the highest standards of practice. That includes the magnet standards of excellence. We have an obligation to the organization, the nursing staff, and our patients to strive to fully integrate the standards in our nursing department."

Finally, we came to appreciate our magnet initiative as a never-ending journey. We had taken important first steps in creating new structures as the foundation for change. Yet we had work to do to strengthen the processes of communication, collaboration, decision making, leadership development, evidence based practice, and resource management to produce the outcomes of excellence to which we aspired.

These insights opened new horizons that broadened our vision of nursing at Middlesex. Our view had been so much narrower at the start of our magnet journey. To clarify our direction, Colleen Smith once again brought us together at a retreat. She extended the invitation to an even wider audience of nurse leaders to frame a new vision. At that retreat we explored the principles of transformational leadership and created a new vision for nursing. *"Nurses at Middlesex Hospital working together to create and sustain a professional practice environment that attracts and retains the highest caliber of professional nursing staff."*

Strengthening the professional practice environment is now the overarching aim of the nursing department. Each year the leadership team evaluates our progress toward achieving specific goals we defined as a leadership team. Staff nurse leaders participate in the process via the nursing councils. Both internal and external forces form the boundaries of our strategic plan. This reinforces our commitment to the organization, the community, and our profession. At present, department priorities derive from four department goals:

1. Enhance RN satisfaction and professionalism
2. Strengthen participative management
3. Strengthen integration of research and evidence-based practice
4. Demonstrably improve patient safety and the quality of care

The Nursing Strategic Plan sets department priorities and defines our agenda for action. It is a dynamic document keeping us focused as we move now from building structure to strengthening processes that are the key to achieving outcomes of excellence.

Central to realizing our vision are the ongoing efforts we are making to continuously nurture relationships and strengthen collaboration across departments and disciplines. Our magnet application had given testimony how employees at Middlesex described themselves as "family." Virtually every example we included reflected the remarkable interdisciplinary and interdepartmental nature of nursing practice at every level of our organization. For example, we had described collaborative efforts between staff nurses and physical therapists to implement a pre-operative class for patients scheduled for joint replacement. Another example showcased our bariatric surgery program, developed by nurses and surgeons with physical therapists, nutritionists, and psychologists, who are now working to become a center of excellence. Other evidence revealed collaborative work across departments to resolve conflicts, address process problems, and improve the quality of care. We view healthy work relationships as a critical factor in producing excellent outcomes of care in our nursing department and as essential to our progress in defining a new vision for nursing.

As accountable leaders, we have instituted a comprehensive plan for evaluation of nursing services that includes publication of an annual report card. It benchmarks our progress in four outcome quadrants: clinical nurse-sensitive measures; functional dimensions such as RN vacancy, retention, and turnover rates, including demographics of the nursing workforce; satisfaction ratings of patients and nurses; and fiscal measures of performance. The Nursing Work Index survey cycle is every two years, which helps us monitor progress in building a strong practice climate. In addition, we have established a baseline measure of decisional control using the Distribution of Authority Scale (Havens & Vasey, 2003) to help us assess the progress of our council model.

LEADERSHIP: THE ESSENTIAL INGREDIENT

Perhaps the most important lesson learned on our magnet journey is the value of strong nursing leadership at every level of practice. A visionary chief nurse executive with the courage to take risks and the integrity to model professional behaviors set a department agenda for transformative action. Central to its success are nurse leaders among the ranks of managers and staff to actualize our vision. As a result, we are investing heavily in succession planning, developing leadership competencies, and cultivating new nurse leaders to lead a new generation of practitioners into the future.

Peer Mentoring and Peer Review Processes

Colleen Smith and the directors agreed to adopt the principles and strategies outlined by Murphy (1996) in *Leadership IQ* during a retreat held in 1999. At that time we completed the Leadership IQ self-assessment to ascertain our individual and collective strengths in each of the eight leadership roles. Since then, we have used that assessment as the basis for establishing peer mentorship relationships to help us grow as leaders. For example, one director formally partnered with another who excelled in the selector role to strengthen her interview and hiring skills. Another director skilled in the connector role mentored a peer who was having difficulty relating to younger staff members. The language of Leadership IQ is now so familiar that we often refer to each other as the "synthesizer" or "negotiator." Now we are working to implement a more systematic peer review process that involves constructive contractual agreements among directors based on the "match" between directors' development goals and Leadership IQ role skills.

Staff Nurse Leaders

One unexpected but welcomed discovery along our magnet journey has been the emergence of new staff nurse leaders. Several nurses have assumed leadership roles on nursing councils at department and unit levels. Magnet Nurse Champions now serve as consultants and mentors to nurses in other organizations seeking magnet designation. Staff nurses lead CQI teams and quality initiatives. Others lead as unit educators and preceptors for nurses in our graduate nurse residency program. Our professional tier advancement program for nurses is designed to encourage and reward their expertise, ongoing professional development, and involvement in organizational life and has motivated many staff nurses to take on leadership roles. We believe it is now our administrative responsibility to develop their competencies as new nurse leaders, so we are taking strategic steps to provide the coaching, resources, and support they need to flourish in their new roles.

A PROGRESS REPORT

CNO Smith ensures that we periodically pause to reflect on our progress and leads us in making "course corrections" when needed to achieve our vision. We continue to conduct formal gap analyses against professional standards. We are making progress in developing needed databases and using valid measures to evaluate all aspects of the practice climate. We are encouraged by results of formal satisfaction and work environment surveys and by benchmarked findings on clinical, functional, and fiscal indicators that reflect department performance.

Informally, we are energized by signs that the *forces of magnetism* at Middlesex Hospital grow stronger by the day. Nurses report that that they have more voice and authority in the organization. The percentage of BSN-prepared and certified nurses has increased, as has the number of nurses involved in the tier advancement program. More nurses are involved in research activities, using best evidence to change practice, and sharing clinical expertise by teaching and developing competencies in each other. Increasingly, nurses are presenting at regional and national conferences and taking on leadership roles in specialty organizations. Here at Middlesex we burst with pride when they present at *Nursing Grand Rounds* and share testimonials of excellence in presenting peer awards for professional performance at our annual meeting. Their growing initiative and assertiveness encourages us and challenges us to nurture their professional growth.

Yet there is still work to do. We continue to make mistakes and to learn from them as a leadership team. For example, we have changed our plans for transitioning the councils to staff nurse leadership to allow more time for leadership development. This was an unpopular move for those councils that had already appointed a staff nurse as chair. At times we have "forgotten" to seek staff nurse feedback, especially in stressful situations, and nurses have challenged us for falling short of our commitment to shared governance. Nurses remind us when we don't follow through and let us know when communication has broken down. They expect visible nurse leaders who see their workload and appreciate the demands on them, even if those situations can't always be changed.

Our nurses have found their voice. We are working to make sure we continue to hear each other. We are striving to discover and capitalize on the power each of us has to become stronger agents of change. Raising a collective voice we believe we can change the world. Our magnet journey has been a long but memorable experience that holds promise for the future. It has given us vision and direction in our quest to transform the nursing department into a rich and rewarding professional practice climate on behalf of nurses and the patients they serve.

DISCUSSION

When reading this story about the journey to magnet status, we see several important themes emerge: having a dream which transforms into a vision that aligns and excites the department, making connections among the staff, and developing and thriving in a learning environment.

As a transformational leader, Colleen Smith used many strategies to achieve magnet status. First, she provided an environment for the staff to develop a vision together. The story clearly demonstrates the development of vision which dreams about a new, better future that is consistent with the mission of the organization (foresight) and is sensitive to external forces (worldview). The story wonderfully illustrates that visions are not static ideas but are alive and are evaluated and revised as needed. The vision to become a magnet hospital aligned the staff and energized them to be innovative, take risks, make changes, and ultimately be successful. Colleen skillfully and persistently created a culture of commitment to the *forces of magnetism*.

A little less obvious in this story, but equally important, is the use of the transformational leadership strategy of self-esteem. Using the principle of the Pygmalion effect (Chapter 2), Colleen set a high expectation for the staff: to become the first magnet hospital in Connecticut at a time when there were fewer than 30 magnet hospitals in the nation. The staff not only lived up to this high expectation but they exceeded it!

Transformational leaders by bringing out the best in others create new leaders. In this story identifying "staff nurse leaders" illustrates this principle. Colleen and the other nurse leaders call forth the leadership in staff and have created formal developmental programs for a much needed and short supply of future leaders.

When using the lens of complexity science to view this story, we see many examples of systematically connecting people and providing the resources for people to share and learn together. As they journeyed the path, they took small, multiple actions to achieve the vision. They were certainly acting on the "edge of complexity" not knowing where they were going specifically, but willing to go anyway. And they took risk, willing to let people experience failures, admit their mistakes, learn from them, and go forth. Colleen role modeled this by admitting the mistakes she made and by having an attitude of "we don't know where this journey will take us but let's try."

Lastly, the story illustrates how this pioneering group of nurse leaders used Leadership IQ as a framework for leadership development. Colleen and her team connected the staff to the "right cause" (achieving magnet hospital status), not because of the prestige but because it was the best thing for patient outcomes. As they journeyed, they solved problems (problem solver role), capitalized on individual leadership strengths in delegated responsibilities (selector role), and evaluated outcomes on an ongoing basis (evaluator role). The story best illustrates the synergizer role that Colleen and Kathleen played to enable them to achieve this important success together.

REFERENCES

Aiken, L. H. (2002). Superior outcomes for magnet hospitals: The evidence base. In M. McClure & A. S. Hinshaw (Eds.). *Magnet hospitals revisited* (pp. 61–81). Washington, DC: American Nurses Publishing Company.

Aiken, L. H., Clarke, S. P., & Sloane, D. M. (2000). Hospital restructuring: Does it adversely affect care and outcomes? *Journal of Nursing Administration, 30* (10), 457–465.

Aiken, L., Clarke, S., Sloane, D. M., Sochalski, J., & Silber, J. (2002). Hospital nurse staffing, patient mortality, nurse burnout, and job dissatisfaction. *Journal of American Medical Association, 288* (16), 1987–1993.

Aiken L. H., & Patrician, P. (2000). Measuring organizational traits of hospitals: The revised nursing work index. *Nursing Research,* 49 (3), 146–153.

Aiken, L. H., Sloane, D. M., Lake, E. T., Sochalski, J., & Weber, A. L. (1999). Organization and outcomes of impatient AIDS care. *Medical Care, 37* (8), 760–772.

Aiken, L. H., Smith, H. L., & Lake, E. T. (1994). Lower Medicare mortality among a set of hospitals known for good nursing care. *Medical Care, 32* (8), 771–787.

American Nurses Credentialing Center Magnet Recognition Program Application Manual (2004). Silver Springs, MD: American Nurses Association.

American Nurses Credentialing Center (2005). Retrieved April 14, 2005, from http://nursingworld.org/ancc/magnet.html.

Estabrooks, C. A., Midodzi, W. K., Cummings, G. G., Ricker, K. L., & Giovannetti, P. (2005). The impact of hospital nursing characteristics on 30-day mortality. *Nursing Research, (5492),* 74–82.

Havens, D. S., & Vasey, J. (2003). Measuring staff nurse decisional involvement: The decisional involvement scale. *Journal of Nursing Administration, 33* (6), 331–336.

Kramer, M., & Hafner, L. (1989). Shared values: Impact on staff nurse job satisfaction and perceived productivity. *Nursing Research, 38,* 172–177.

Lake, E. T. (2002). Development of the practice environment scale of the nursing work index. *Research in Nursing & Health, 25,* 176–188.

Laschinger, H. K., Almost, J., & Tuer-Hodes, D. (2003). Workplace empowerment and magnet hospital characteristics. *Journal of Nursing Administration, 33* (7/8), 410–422.

McClure, M., & Poulin, M., & Sovie, M. D. (1983). *Magnet hospitals: Attraction and retention of professional nurses.* American Academy of Nursing Task Force on Nursing Practice in Hospitals. Kansas City, MO: American Nurses Association.

McClure, M. L., & Hinshaw, A. S. (Eds.). (2002). *Magnet hospitals revisited.* Washington, DC: American Nurses Publishing.

Murphy, E. (1996). *Leadership IQ.* New York: John Wiley & Sons.

Scott, J. G., Sochalski, J., & Aiken, L. (1999). Review of magnet hospital research. *Journal of Nursing Administration, 29* (1), 9–19.

Stolzenberger, K. (2003). Beyond the award: The ANCC magnet program as the framework for culture change. *Journal of Nursing Administration, 33* (10), 522–531.

Upenieks, V. (2002). Assessing differences in job satisfaction of nurses in magnet and nonmagnet hospitals. *Journal of Nursing Administration, 32* (11), 564–576.

CHAPTER 17

Complexity Science in Action

Linda Rusch

INTRODUCTION

This chapter is the personal account of how complexity science can revolutionize the work environment, moving from a system of control and rigid authority to viewing the organization through the lens of complexity. Before reading this chapter, you may want to review some of the basic concepts of complexity science in Chapter 5.

THE HUNTERDON MEDICAL CENTER STORY

Hunterdon Medical Center (HMC) is a not-for-profit 180-bed facility. Part of the Hunterdon Healthcare System, it is located in Flemington, New Jersey. More than 50 years ago Flemington was a rural county of 46,000 people with 25 medical practitioners. A vision of HMC inspired by Dr. E. Corwin brought about—not only a hospital—but also a model medical center and an integrated system of health care services. General practitioners automatically became admitted to the attending staff of the hospital. Community need determined the choice of specialists. Concurrently, HMC founders began an affiliation with a medical school. Some unique relationships began.

Right from the beginning, community members stepped forward with human and financial resources. They raised more than $1.2 million. Seventy-five percent of Flemington's citizens contributed to the fund-raising campaign at a time when the average annual income was approximately $3,500 a year. Volunteer recruitment got underway. From this collective community effort, the medical center manifested what many called the "miracle in the cornfield."

Today Hunterdon Medical Center continues to care for its communities by providing acute care as well as preventative care.

What makes this community hospital so special? To answer this, come along with me.

The hospital sits up on a hill, far enough from the main road to look quite vast. Well-manicured lawns and seasonal flowers and shrubs always add just enough color to complement the setting. To mitigate parking challenges presented by growth of services, HMC offers valet parking free of charge. As one parks and approaches the main entrance, a medium-sized man with a slight southern drawl and a big smile greets every person. His sincere offers of "May I help you?" "Good morning," or "Have a good day" provide just the tonic most of us need to start the day.

HMC's hospital community has a remarkable feel unlike many other medical center facilities. Visitors and new employees particularly take notice of this. Some have described it as an aura, an energy, a good karma, and definitely palpable.

Hunterdon manifests all that and more. During the past 10 years the nursing department has had a 97.5 percent retention rate and also has scored in the 90s for patient satisfaction in nursing. In a 2002 survey employee satisfaction ranked higher than 95 percent. The employees appear exceptionally friendly, helpful, and very proud. Employees have a collective consciousness to excel voluntarily. A culture of commitment reigns.

So what is complexity science in action?

The phrase *complexity science* describes an emerging field that examines living systems. The science looks at how systems actually behave, rather than how they should behave. It invites leaders to examine the unpredictable, disorderly and chaotic aspects of their organizations. In unveiling a complex picture, it gives added dimension and complements our traditional understanding of organizations. The study of complexity science brings added insight to visualize and understand organizations. In a nonlinear interactive manner, it discloses emergent properties, continuous change, and unpredictable outcomes.

Veteran health care leaders can find themselves frustrated by increasingly new and fast-paced, chaotic and complex environments. Traditional methods of leadership often prove ineffective. Existing organizational leadership paradigms grew out of a decision-making tradition from Newtonian physics. These leaders by training and expectation predict outcomes. Complexity science, on the other hand, teaches that controlling, planning, and decision-making work in stable environments, not in unstable chaotic environments.

At HMC each patient care unit embraces the differences from the clinical service line, and from the uniqueness of the people working interdependently on that unit. The leader works as an integral part of each unit.

On most days, while walking through the units, one often hears laughter. An air of collaboration resides within. Team members reflect the high-functioning qualities of acknowledgment and respect for one another. This dance has a rhythm, energy, and fun that pervades the hospital community. One senses an unspoken motto of "No matter what, we can do this." On the other hand, days also may occur when the team does not reflect a high-performing, collaborative, and friendly air. Instead, they may show fatigue, irritability, and stress. Organizations, after all, have dynamic, ever-changing, and largely unpredictable properties.

As the chief nursing officer of Hunterdon Medical Center, I have had the good fortune of studying complexity science. I believe this science has helped me be a more effective transformational leader.

Complexity science reframes our view of how social systems behave. It teaches us to observe different patterns of behavior and that these patterns provide insights into sustainability and vitality of organizations.

The example I gave regarding a group of staff not functioning always at its peak reminds us that human beings comprise systems. All their interactive relationships affect the group, both positively and negatively. They do not function as a machine.

The machine metaphor has serious limitations when applied to humans. Clearly, humans have so much more than programmed machine parts; the reflect dynamic swings of energy and interactiveness from negative to positive and vice versa.

New outcomes of behavior emerge from systems made up of humans. Complex health care delivery systems have highly interdependent relationships. A change in one part of the system can have tremendous effects, negative or positive, on other parts of the systems.

No single person working at Hunterdon Medical Center knows the workings of Hunterdon Medical Center, and yet collectively Hunterdon Medical Center acts and performs. Often one can observe that during a crisis people come together of their own accord; order replaces chaos for free.

Leading with a lens of "living systems," as opposed to a machine lens, brings comfort and hope. Using the lens of nature and/or living systems provides an excellent start for transforming health care delivery. Both share the goal of survival.

I present my own experience, by way of example, for how I lead with a complexity science lens.

I have served as Hunterdon Medical Center's chief nursing officer for 13 years; I can honestly say I look forward to going to work. Relationships provide the key element. They support and energize me. By means of relationships,

I connect with others around common purposes. I care deeply about the staff, the patients, and community members with and for whom I work.

My role involves "sense making." Living in a largely unpredictable and unknowing world, we often encounter systems and experience new and unfamiliar frontiers. The landscape is rugged. A transformational leader has to make sense out of this rugged landscape. The leader makes sense by looking, observing, analyzing, asking questions, and noting new patterns that emerge. This often takes place in collaboration with other people and their respective realities. Ready-made answers do not apply to new frontiers.

Health care workers today have enormous knowledge. They deserve meaningful work, and the feeling of making a difference. They must have involvement in the sense-making process.

HMC has had a shared governance professional practice model since 1990. This model gives nursing a very necessary voice to transform health care. Overprescribing or micromanaging does not produce transformational change. Even if one does not have a shared governance model, any system that gives nursing and other employees a voice will work. No one person has control—not even the chief nursing officer. We have, as do the other players, an influence on the system. Control represents an illusion. As chief nursing officer you do not have control, no one does. It is an illusion. Consequently, we all come across those some label as "resistors." I highlight the word *resistor* because the word carries a negative connotation. We may fail to see the good that they may contribute.

Think of these resistors as people who prefer different patterns of behavior. To help an organization change you must understand the active attractors and work with them in order to move to different and more complex problems. Having people with different mental models often allows new ideas to emerge.

In complexity science the greater the diversity and the more robust, the more likely it is for creative ideas to emerge, particularly when you want to implement a new process. For example, you can create a conversation around, "How would a new health care delivery system look where nurses thrive and patients receive quality patient/family centered safe care?"

Nursing councils resemble trees. Councils provide a context for sharing information, developing relationships, connecting and inviting people to partner in co-creating the future. Formal roles in an organization do not explain the whole or how things get done. Relationships create change and people thrive behind the formal structures of organizational charts and reporting lines.

Some have called me a "butterfly," cross-pollinating information, stories, praise from one area of the system to another; this very act can influence and shape outcomes. The lens of complexity science also helps me understand that small changes can have big effects and big changes can often make no difference.

Approximately two years ago a number of us set out to influence a change in the culture to help create an environment of patient safety. Rather than a top-down approach, we used an upside-down approach, by going to staff at the "sharp end" in their world and asking questions about how they felt about safety: "What is not working?" "What is broken?"

Powerful stories ensued. Our language supported their stories for greater sharing, encouragement, and truth. Did I forget to mention that you have to want to know the truth?

Complex adaptive systems always include elements of surprise. For example, you experience this any time your day as planned does not go the way you intended. Much like in nature, you encounter surprise and serendipity.

Using the metaphor of planning a garden, you may begin with a vision of how it might look. You create a good-enough plan; you nurture the garden by watering, fertilizing, and weeding. Something beautiful results from your labor. You will not get it right in advance; design is ongoing, dynamic, and unfolding. People make up organizations in a largely unpredictable and unknowing world. Consider how fast new information arrives, and how change affects our lives. The notion "I do not know" versus "I know" frees me to work in groups and teams with diversified thoughts, ideas, and brilliance.

One morning at 7:30 a.m. I attended a patient safety action team meeting. It consisted of diverse players from different departments, different management levels, and nonmanagement staff members. I heard laughter. I observed a willingness to work together. I felt the energy of creative ideas unleashed.

When a team diversifies, no hierarchy becomes imposed. All contribute and you witness genuine respect and collaboration. I have personally witnessed this more than a hundred times. Leaders who do all the talking, and do not ask questions, or who do not help create the environment, miss the point when the dance occurs. The power of relationships emerges.

If you contemplate any type of cultural shift, you should involve as many staff members as possible. This diversity provides the energy for change. As part of the system yourself, you must accept the possibility of transformation. You learn as you go.

You improvise, like a great jazz ensemble. You have just enough min specs, or a good-enough plan, to give you some directives. So how do you use min specs? You can use this process to encourage self-organization rather than to impose top-down compliance. Min specs might include elements of a mission statement, guiding principles, etc. Allow space for possible change. If you pay attention, new ideas or "surprises" emerge.

Stay with me. Walk along with me down the corridors. What do you see, hear, smell, and sense?

Use the lens of human nature. It involves more than just seeing. Instead, you are centered, focused, present, and alert enough to pay attention to the interaction of others. Bring this experience to your own place of work. Shadow your staff and discover the remarkable and amazing new environment.

Be comfortable with ambiguity. The amount of ambiguity relates directly to the amount of leadership required. Days will occur when you will wonder how to do your job. Healthy organizations exhibit a certain degree of chaos as leaders try to make sense of it and deal with the ambiguity.

A number of years ago I asked all nurse leaders and staff nurse council members what it would look like if nurses cared for their community. I wanted to encourage the nurses to make changes where they felt they could. Small changes resemble drops of rain falling in a still pond. This small change can create a ripple effect, replicating and spreading throughout the system. In line with this vision, I attached the following to the concept: (1) any nurse can take off up to a half-day per pay period to work on a community health initiative outside the hospital; (2) do not do anything illegal; (3) take the funds out of a limited outreach budget on your own, and let the other members of the group know what you are doing.

Within weeks I learned of 27 different initiatives started by various nurses who wanted to do something. We created the conditions so that nurses who wanted to do something could do it. The experiences involved addressing issues of domestic violence, women's shelters, food for the homeless, health fairs, and public education seminars. I think they always will remember this experience. Six of the projects took on a life of their own by receiving support from the organization for further growth.

So how did this work?

We had a good-enough vision, nurses caring for their community. We did not get bogged down with over prescription or detail. We had intrinsic motivation—"attractor patterns" of just enough interest to get going. Finally, we had our simple rules, just enough boundaries, and opportunities for everyone to use their 15 percent influence in the system.

To this day I hear many new stories regarding nurses reaching out to their community. The staff continues to give from the heart.

Are we paying enough attention to relationships?

In my opinion, divisions, functions, departments, units, teams, cliques, in-groups and out-groups often make-up teams, a social system. Relationships then can represent either assets or debits.

As leaders, we have a tremendous opportunity to capitalize on our human capital by focusing on the concept of "human-centered organizations." Whereas structure and control accompany simple machine-like situations, our new world involves instead communication, cooperation, collaboration, and trust, necessary components for successful organizations to survive, prosper, learn, and adapt.

Continue to walk with me.

We notice the director of maternity walking briskly up the hall. As she passes, she informs me that in her very full unit, "Babies are popping out all over." Since no one on the staff had time for a lunch break, the director of nursing ordered pizza. She goes on to say that they shared the pizza with pediatrics, another very busy unit that day.

On another morning the night supervisor smiled and exclaimed, "Bringing in those massage therapists over the weekend was a great idea; the staff was thrilled," another example of caring and concern.

The entire staff works hard. You care for your staff by recognizing their feelings, beliefs, passion, and ideas. Nurture them as you would nurture your garden. If we fail to care, we can anticipate the same outcomes as a neglected garden.

Let me add a few more favorite concepts: Benoit Mandlebrot (1977), who discovered fractal geometry, explained how self-similarity exhibits identical or similar patterns on different scales. For example, take a tree with its branching patterns, or the branching structure of the lung, all the way to the alveoli. Organizations also have this self-similarity. Healthy leaders have healthy staff. I once heard at a conference about a group of chief nursing officers who presented a session about imbalance with their jobs. As a result of long hours, little sleep, little exercise, and eating poorly, their lives began to fall apart. They experienced mental, physical, and spiritual decline. Once the chief nursing officers made real changes and became healthier, their directors, their staff, and the other executives also became healthier. A noticeable shift occurred.

Let's go back to the illustration of nurses who care for their community. This is another example of self-similarity. Generally, healthy hospitals reside in healthy communities. Healthy families belong to healthy communities. And along the same lines individuals reside in healthy families. Communities need healthy environments, organizations, and associations that nurture everyone. Finally, society nurtures communities by recognizing the importance of each person.

Do we have influence?

Most people have about 15 percent control over their work situation. The other 85 percent are organizationally imposed structures and systems over which you have no control. Fifteen percent may seem small, but that 15 percent has allowed us to accomplish a great deal in a nonlinear, complex adaptive system. As nurses we have heard that homeostasis is a good thing. We now realize this concept of status quo/homeostasis also can indicate a death sentence. Certain attractor patterns can become traps. To be alive, dynamic, and adaptable, we need a certain amount of chaos. A remarkable change sometimes can occur as a result of this 15 percent.

In 2004 the latest Institute of Medicine (IOM) report came out entitled "Transforming the Work Environment of Nurses: Keeping Patients Safe." I read this 400-plus page document with great interest and passion and was committed to use this book. I wanted this report to be a stimulus for the future. Not wanting to pursue this task alone, I asked nurse directors to read the book, and they in turn asked their interested staff nurses to also read it. Each director and their staff took one chapter for review and analysis. The teams then made their own assessments of their environments and included recommendations. Staff and directors also took time outside of work and at several off-site locations to produce with pride a final report.

Six months later the Hunterdon Medical Center nursing department had its own IOM report. We acknowledged our patients and everyone who worked on it. We shared the document with almost 50 groups, wanting to hear other recommendations and suggestions related to both sustainability and implementation. The process brought attention to creating conditions for self-organization, rather than a more traditional, top-down approach. Collectively, we witnessed the formation of generative relationships.

We deemphasized notions of knowing in advance and focused more on tuning in to the environment, sense making, and building on "what works." In addition to involvement of numerous groups and the diffusion of information, complexity science teaches us that multiple actions help. They encourage participants to try a number of different actions and see what arises rather than insisting on certainty or having it fail-safe before beginning this exploration. Complexity science calls this "hunting and gathering." Nurse directors began to ask their staff members: "What do nurses hunt and gather for? How much time do nurses spend working in broken systems? Could nurses become more effective healers if they did not have to run at staccato pace?" Nurses then talked about system failure.

The nurses had wonderful, visceral reactions to having their directors ask them these questions. No one had ever asked about such things before. Just the mere asking of the question brought hope. Broken systems, as we discussed, have a way of staying broken until we initiate some sort of change. And often just asking questions and having conversations can lead to a shift. At just about the same time, the practice council compiled its own list of system improvement recommendations and began inviting staff from different departments to discuss change to improve the system for patient care.

The single action of reviewing the IOM report led to multiple actions. As we shape and respond to new ideas and actions, the change itself shapes us much more than simply causing us to adapt to external change. We call this co-creating. As the number of connections between people increases, the outcomes of these connections grow. Again, even though you may have planned ahead, you can always count on surprises. The hunting-and-gathering questions and resulting process of engagement have become so rich that we do it on an ongoing basis.

So, how far on the edge do you want to be?

All organizations need a balance. Clockware and swarmware must dance together. By clockware I mean all the things with which one has to comply or exercise control—JCAHO, Department of Health, OSHA, CMS, policies, etc. However, out of control swarmware really does bring about adaptability. Creativity and survival need spontaneous learning networks with open conflict and dialogue. They remain vital for living systems (us). They remain very close to the edge of chaos where things appear loose and fluid. So how much swarmware do we have in our organization? Well, the elements of chaos include a tension between order and chaos. Take a look at your meeting structures. Do opportunities exist for open dialogue and conflict? Does anyone ask those wicked questions that expose paradox?

What would it be like if meetings were exciting, free flowing, and creative?

Clockware suggests a certain formality needed to get the job done or get through an agenda. Nevertheless, as a leader, try to allow enough time to connect to those relationships. At our nurse management meetings, we have two agenda items that allow for some swarmware to occur. We call these "House Issues" and "Lessons Learned." The first item allows anyone to discuss any issue they want. Very often this conversation becomes intense. Different viewpoints emerge. These sessions often include comments of appreciation about the process. The leader must provide this unstructured open space and unpredictable portion of the agenda that allows spontaneous dialogue to emerge. At the same time the leader also must create a safe, protective environment to encourage open, honest, and creative reflection. These conversations, while allowing for support, can trigger creative innovations that probably would not occur by following a standard agenda.

As leaders we set a context to celebrate and learn from both success and failure. We know we learn through failures. Anyone who makes a mistake has done a favor to the organization if it leads to organizational learning and change.

At Hunterdon Medical Center we have a "no blame culture." Anyone can write up a medication error report, even an anonymous one. We give nurses who come forward an angel stickpin as a reward. We thank people who come forward. We think about our language. You often hear the expression, "There are no bad people, but there are bad systems." We know that very few people get up in the morning with the intent to mess up their organizations. Sometimes it's the complicated processes and distractions that lead to mistakes. With this culture of "no blame," we have witnessed a remarkable increase in reporting of med errors at level 1. Level 1 med errors are potential medication errors intercepted by a nurse before they reach the patient. Reporting these helps us to create better systems for our patients.

Let's examine in a little more detail the notion of leadership and the 15 percent influence.

No leader can affect more than 15 percent of the things around her. Knowledge of this has freed us from the common illusion that we are in control and has resulted in less anxiety. We have influence, but we do not control everything. Just imagine, however, if each person on your team used his 15 percent toward a common vision.

More than two years ago we introduced computer charting for nursing. True to form, the staff went through the new procedures with flying colors. They had adaptable and resilient attitudes. Why? Because they had meaningful involvement from the planning stage right on to choosing the type of computer, which they fondly call their "buddy." Remember every change has a technical and social aspect. If we do not handle well the social human aspects of change, the technically rational changes can fail.

Through listening, observing, and hearing the nurse stories, we have entered the world of technology with computers, wireless phones, faxes, high tech beds, four channel pumps, PCAs, new modalities, new supervision, new intervention, and new everything. High tech has arrived. In different ways than previously, nurses try to balance their fast-paced staccato lives of doing more than 160 tasks in eight hours.

What can we do as leaders to help preserve the essence of caring?

The IOM report "Crossing the Quality Chasm" provides a strategy and action plan for building a stronger system during the next decade. Without being overly prescriptive, it asks for innovation at the local level. It also advances 10 simple rules to guide the patient-clinician relationship in the 21st century. For example, it mentions using the healing relationship as a basis for care. The high touch culture can balance the high tech.

If we have only 15 percent influence, then think if we all had a common vision, a vision where we would create with others a healing environment for patients and an environment that was safe without needless errors or death. This environment would include nurses as healing coaches who care for patients and families in mutually gratifying ways.

Complexity science offers us many insights on how to lead in a health care environment that needs transformation. You as a leader can join with your directors and staff to create a shared vision. This shared vision provides a force of power that produces a common identity and a commitment to move people to a new attractor.

At Hunterdon Medical Center, the journey has begun toward the vision of "creating an environment where nurses thrive." Out of this vision has emerged another profound vision of having "nurses become healing coaches." The balance of high technology with high touch (caring) has become a major focus. We listen to conversations in nonjudgmental ways. We observe the patterns that emerge. We experiment. We push the boundaries so that we do not remain status quo. We cross-pollinate with information and stories. We allow open space for creative ideas to emerge. We acknowledge that organizations have messy and noisy components. We appreciate that informal relationships, gossip, and even rumors contribute to perception and actions.

We do not have all the answers, nor do we know the exact direction to go. Great changes with lots of fanfare do not produce transformation. We can begin to transform the health care delivery system, with the help of others. We know that change is fundamentally based on the interaction of relationships. Because we live in a complex adaptive system where possibilities thrive and anything can happen, this should give us hope for the future.

If all health care leaders would read the latest IOM report "Keeping Patients Safe: Transforming the Work Environment of Nurses" and create a shared vision, we then could start to have a conversation with our staff about this. Form small groups of early adaptors. Link these groups together with other groups and spread information. Let the system emerge over time. Emerging behavior will look different in all of our organizations because the cultures are different. But think of the novelty and the number of new and different experiments taking hold. All this diversity and creativity can help us learn how to provide a safe and healing environment for our patients, nurses, and other practitioners.

So do you want to come along for the ride?

I welcome you to come along for the ride. It makes no difference what metaphor is more comfortable and to your liking. Whether it is skiing down a mountain and executing the surprise moguls with great finesse or galloping through beautiful meadows on a horse only to be surprised by a swarm of bees, this life is full of adventure and opportunity.

Hold on, take the reigns, and be prepared for the ride of a lifetime!

Once you come to accept the messy and sometimes scary world we live in, and realize it is alive with opportunity, you can relax and go with nature's flow. You cannot stop the river; the river flows on its own. It has its own force.

As chief nursing officer, how I show up constitutes my most important contribution. When I am centered, present, and alert, I can be aware of all the fabulous relationships that I am a part of. I cherish the fact that I take part in a system we refer to as "human systems."

Being authentic and vulnerable allows me to be more human, and being more human allows me to enter into relationships more fully. Knowing I am not alone on this journey never traveled is very comforting. So much brilliance and creativity can occur when a group comes together. I am constantly amazed at the potential ideas and solutions that emerge with the connectivity of people. I understand deeply that this very connectedness with others calls forth from us a tremendous sense of commitment and purpose to do good things.

Remember that your own personal development leads to organizational development. This is crucial. For if you do not take risks, live on the edge at times by pushing the boundaries, experimenting with new concepts or ideas, not only will you be part of homeostasis but so will your followers.

We all have that 15 percent influence on our systems. Let us begin collectively to try some small changes. We may be surprised at what a huge revolution may occur in health care.

DISCUSSION

This account about complexity science is a beautiful example of the whole being more than the sum of its parts. It shows the humanness of being a leader while demonstrating how complexity science, transformational leadership, and leadership IQ work seamlessly and in concert to actualize the role competencies of the leader. Although written by a chief nursing officer, the theory and many of the examples are about clinical units and can be applied by any clinical leader in any setting at any level of the organization.

This story not only illustrates every major concept of complexity science described in Chapter 5, but it takes the concepts to the next level, application to practice. The definition of complexity science in Chapter 5 states, "When viewing the world from the perspective of complexity science, it is composed of many *complex adaptive systems* that are nonlinear systems in which diverse agents interact with each other and are capable of undergoing spontaneous *self-organization.* Within these complex adaptive systems, *relationships and connectedness* between the agents in the systems are the most important components of the system rather than individual agents. Complex adaptive systems are *embedded* in one another and are ever-changing and adaptable; thus, the world is fundamentally *unpredictable* and *uncontrollable.* Yet from this apparent *disorder arise order and patterns* that are governed by *simple rules.*

Linda's account illustrates clearly that Hunterdon Medical Center is a *complex adaptive system (CAS)* in which are *embedded* other CASs, clinical units and human beings to name a few. In addition, the medical center is *embedded* in the Flemington community and is thus responsive to its local environment. Throughout the story Linda stresses the *importance of relationships and connecting* diverse people and the role of the leader in doing this. She clearly shows how the organization is *uncontrollable and unpredictable,* but most important, her acceptance that "control is an illusion," has energized her and the staff to be creative, take risks, accept and learn from failures in order to learn, grow, and be successful. Using *simple rules* ("min specs"), she provides a "good-enough" vision that then allows for self-organization. Last, she demonstrates that among the chaos, *patterns emerge,* there is order, and from this the medical center is thriving.

Clearly, Linda is a transformational leader, but more important she is nurturing and developing her clinical leaders to be transformational leaders as well. She has developed an organization based on trust and on bringing out the best in everybody. Her story is peppered with examples of visionary leadership. But the best example of this is how she has learned about, embraced, and is living complexity science, demonstrating an extraordinary skill in being visionary and developing visionary leaders. She has viewed the organization through the lens of complexity and has institutionalized it throughout Hunterdon.

Linda also demonstrates many of the principles of Leadership IQ. She is an exemplary *connector,* connecting the staff to the right causes such as community involvement and patient safety. She is a *problem solver* because first and foremost she is willing to listen and find the problems. Her statement, "Did I forget to mention that you have to want to know the truth?" clearly demonstrates her willingness to identify and solve problems. And most of all Linda is clearly a *synergizer,* motivating and enabling the staff to achieve improvement together.

Although not asked to address role competencies in her story, she has provided examples of most of them. The story cannot be told about complexity science and transformational leadership without concrete, real-world achievements and outcomes. To name a few, we point out that Linda has passionately pursued putting together a system to improve patient safety, she is community and consumer focused, and she has marketed the nursing department to the community.

To conclude I would like to point out some additional important issues discussed in this book that this story illustrates. First, the history of the medical center and its birth and growth provide a unique mission and important story that aligns the staff to fulfill the mission. Second, although not an emphasis in the story, Linda sees the organization as a system of microsystems with each patient care unit defining itself by the clinical service line (subpopulations of patients) and by the people working on that unit. Third, her story is rich in descriptive language, a technique that helps people understand the vision. She uses metaphors such as "dancing," "growing gardens," and "playing jazz," for instance. Finally, this staff laughs and has fun!

REFERENCES

Mandelbrot, B. B. (1977). *Fractals: Form, chance and dimension*. San Francisco: W. H. Freeman and Company.

Index

Note: Page numbers followed by "t" denote tables